ALMOST CONSISTENT FITNESS

BOB MULLIGAN, PhD

AN EASY HABIT RESET
NO PERFECTION, NO STRESS & ONE SIMPLE RULE

~~ALMOST~~ CONSISTENT FITNESS

THE SECRET OF HOW TO MAKE

FITNESS WALKING

YOUR CONSISTENCY SOLUTION

*INCLUDES A 12-WEEK TRACKER

BOB MULLIGAN, PhD

Almost Consistent Fitness © copyright 2025 by Bob Mulligan. All rights reserved. No part of this book may be reproduced in any form whatsoever, by photography or xerography or by any other means, by broadcast or transmission, by translation into any kind of language, nor by recording electronically or otherwise, without permission in writing from the author, except by a reviewer, who may quote brief passages in critical articles or reviews.

The Fitness Success Promotions Group, LLC
San Diego-Denver-St.Croix

ISBNs: 979-8-218-61525-3 (pbk); 979-8-218-55600-6 (ebook)

Cover and book design byMolly Mortimer, Mayfly book design

Library of Congress Catalog Number: 2024924329
First Printing: 2025

CONTENTS

Intro 1

F.itness A.ttitude T.raining 19

Self-Sabotage, Barriers, and Traps. 41

Think Habits. 61

Think Process, Not Goals. 69

Find the Perfect Coach. 74

The Fundamental Principle for Success Is "Just Show Up." 79

The Walking Breakthrough. 85

Walking Strategies—A Practical Guide. 101

Getting Your S**** Together... The Plan. 119

My Fitness Commitment. 123

The Almost Consistent Fitness Streak Tracker. 125

12-Week Almost Consistent Fitness Streak Tracker 137

Acknowledgments 189

INTRO

> "If at first you don't succeed, skydiving is not for you."
>
> —Steven Wright

Has your exercise routine been hit or miss, inconsistent, or missing in action? If so, you've probably tried more than once to get it back. Maybe you made a resolution and got some gear, shoes, equipment, or a membership pass to a gym.

You were all fired up. You envisioned yourself as a lean, mean fighting machine.

Then you missed a day the first week. Two the next. In the third week, you managed to work out once. And not once since.

The major frustration is simply this: you've been fit before, maybe even an athlete, and have enjoyed the benefits of exercise, but for one reason or another, you're just unable to lock in and get it going again.

You're starting to see a pattern of inconsistent exercise, and to put it mildly, you're pissed. And you're also starting to put some pretty ugly labels on your behavior. Like you're a No-Hoper or worse.

It becomes increasingly clear that getting in shape is the easy part; staying in shape is the tough part. Like the *Seinfeld* episode, "Anyone can take a reservation; it's holding the reservation, that's the important part!"

Well, relax. It's not nearly as grim as you think. In my experience working with thousands of folks over many years, I've found that most people who struggle to stick with their fitness program are just making a few easily correctable mistakes.

Success is much closer than you imagine with a shift in attitude, a change in focus, and, most importantly, a system to help you move around the barriers and inevitable roadblocks.

With a systematic approach that promotes consistency over short-term results, success is possible and probable.

Does this mean that if you follow this process, you will have attained fitness perfection for the rest of your life? Probably not.

Typically, there are inevitable slip-ups, but when you stumble in the future, you'll have the tools to get back up and self-correct.

By the way, you're not alone: about 40% of the US population falls into a category referred to as the on-again/off-again or the inconsistent exerciser. These folks know the benefits; they want to be fit again, but for various reasons, they struggle. That's the category you undoubtedly fall into. After all, you're reading this book and will likely have concluded . . . it's time!

So what about the other 60%? Let's take a minute to review all the categories to be certain you're in the right one.

According to a health club industry survey several years ago, the three categories are as follows.

THE SUCCESSFUL: THE FIT AND ACTIVE.

Roughly 20% of the population is engaged in a regular fitness activity; they're Fit and Active.

Remember that many in the Fit and Active group struggled with consistency for some time, and then, something clicked. They found a strategy that worked. They've learned to love the process and take pride in their ongoing success, but they don't take it for granted.

This book is all about trying to get you into that category. I'm in that category, and it's a good place to be.

An impressive subgroup in the Fit and Active group has never struggled. They enjoyed the challenge of fitness from the jump. They look at the book's title and seem puzzled. What do you mean by *almost* consistent fitness? You either do it or you don't. And if you do it, you do it the right way, push hard, and enjoy the process. It's all about discipline and willpower. They don't get us!

This book is not for them. I have several friends in this category.

THE DISINTERESTED: THE NO-HOPERS.

This second category encompasses 40% of the population, and it is a complete flip of the previous Fit and Active category: the No-Hopers. No-Hopers have no interest in becoming fit. Zero. And by self-identification, they are No-Hopers.

There's some ebb and flow between these categories. A No-Hoper may have a come-to-Jesus moment and begin an incredible fitness journey. But the odds of that happening are like winning the lottery—beyond rare.

The great thing about most No-Hopers is that they're very clear on their position regarding exercise. They'll give you a laugh, and the most typical comment is, "Not a chance." I have several friends in this category.

Trust me, No-Hopers are not interested in this book. However, if you self-identify as a No-Hoper but are slightly intrigued by the title, well... maybe you're a borderline Hoper. If so, welcome.

THE INCONSISTENT AND FRUSTRATED EXERCISERS: THE HOPERS.

Then there's the remaining 40%. I call them the Hopers. This is just rough math, but in that 30 to 59-year-old demographic, there are somewhere around 60 to 70 million Hopers. Mostly, these people want to exercise but haven't been able to do so consistently for one reason or another. This is the group I've spent my life's work helping.

This book is aimed at the incredibly large population of on-again-off-again exercisers. This group tends to be full of life; they want to extract it all. They want a practical approach to fitness, a doable and hopefully enjoyable part of the long and healthy life they imagine.

I can see it when I talk to them about the possibilities of restarting their program. They intellectually understand the benefits of exercise. Unfortunately, they've gotten caught up in a cycle of ineffective strategies and don't understand some pretty simple work-arounds or fixes. In so many subtle and not-so-subtle ways, they've sabotaged themselves. On top of all that, they've become somewhat commitment-phobic.

If I had to put my finger on the nature of their commitment-phobia, it would be perfectionism—particularly amongst former athletes who remember their desire to push themselves through the discomfort to get as close to the threshold of perfection as possible.

Well, healthy, moderate fitness is a different game, and you might be letting *perfection* get in the way of *pretty good*. The program we present is all about moving from frustration and inaction to pretty good.

Longevity expert Dr. Peter Attia reports on current research demonstrating dramatic benefits from exercise, even at relatively modest levels. Going from zero to moderate, consistent exercise is golden.

It turns out that pretty good is not all that bad.

With you in mind, I'll show you a plan with a few practical steps, including one simple strategy that you can use to transform your frustration into an ultimate breakthrough.

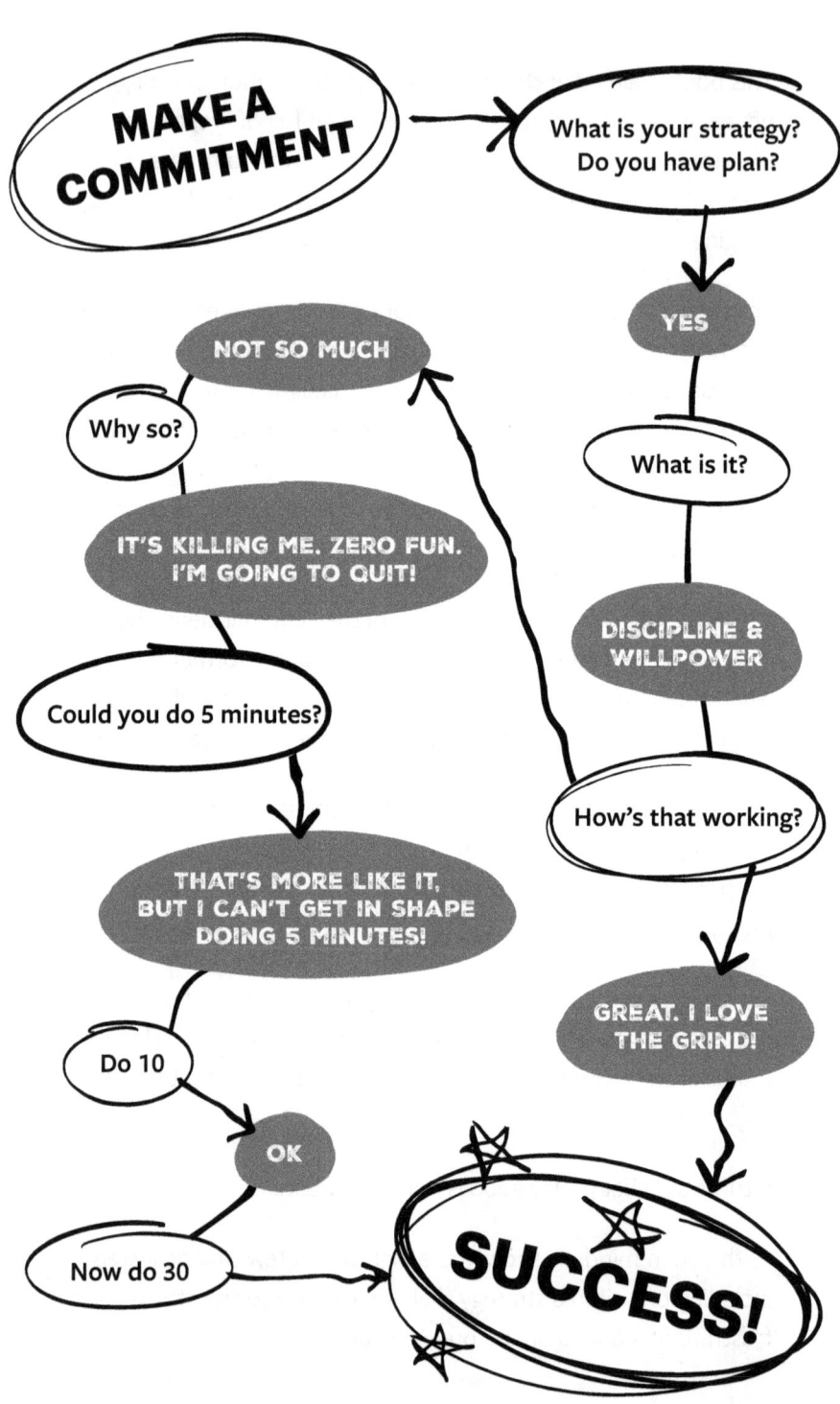

In the world of sports performance, a breakthrough is an ability or skill the athlete discovers through trial and error or with the benefit of some coaching. And it's typically something they already possess. They, in effect, unleash a superpower from within.

The plan's premise is simple: Establish a daily habit of intentional, scheduled movement—an activity that's so easy and accessible that it will be hard to refuse.

My commitment is to help you get going again in a physical activity. You may even have one you'd like to return to, and I'm good with that.

But let me explain why walking—one simple, doable, yet surprisingly effective exercise—might be your best choice, foundation, and ultimate answer.

World-class powerlifting legend Mark Bell said it all when talking about the best possible fitness foundation you could have, "If you can stay connected to one thing, if you can stay tethered to one habit, I would say walking would be a great place to start."

Once you've established fitness walking as your platform, you can always add other fitness activities, knowing that you can return to your simple, solid walking routine at the first sign of struggle.

Your foundational walking habit will keep your consistent fitness streak alive. It will always be there for you.

WHY IS INTENTIONAL FITNESS WALKING THE BEST ACTIVITY?

> "There is so much life to live, and if you just keep on breathing and keep on walking, you will get through everything."
>
> —Brian Welsh

Brisk walking is rich in health benefits. A daily walking program produces biochemical changes in the body, from improvements in the heart and circulatory system to reductions in anxiety and depression, reduced dementia risk, and the burning of extra calories.

But maybe the stat that jumps off the page is from a 2021 study reported in *JAMA* which shows that people who've logged at least 7,000 steps per day have a 50 to 70% lower risk of premature death compared to those who walked fewer than 7,000 steps per day.

And walking adds one more giant plus.

With the right approach and a little time, you'll find it becoming something you look forward to, something that becomes indispensable and—dare I say—enjoyable.

You may choose to include strength training in your routine, and I hope you do, but walking will be your rock, your foundation. You need something with a high do-ability rating, and walking is all of that and more. It's the ultimate excuse destroyer.

You'll fight for your right to walk; you won't let them take it away. You'll respect the walk.

How important can walking be to your success? If you put me in a situation and told me my life depended on you successfully maintaining a healthy, lifelong, consistent fitness program, I would choose walking!

But don't get me wrong. If you give walking a shot, a fair chance, and feel it's not your thing, you may have some other activity you've done in the past, like biking or swimming or whatever. I'm good with that.

After all, the primary focus of this book is to help you develop a daily habit of movement. Learn to avoid the roadblocks and barriers we face and get activity back into your life.

I'm thrilled as long as your Daily Motion Detector registers on the high side.

THE SPORTS PSYCHOLOGY OF FITNESS.

> "Pavlov, that name sure rings a bell."
>
> —Don Fridley

I've been influenced in my career by the work of legendary psychologists such as B.F. Skinner or Albert Bandura, as well as the work of contemporary scientists and authors like Katy Milkman, Wendy Wood, Michelle Segar, Judson Brewer, James Clear, Mark Manson, BJ Fogg and Ryan Holiday. However, most of the inspiration for this book comes from the athletic fields—the basketball courts and the golf courses.

Specifically, the labs of applied modern sports psychology. Current examples of applying these principles are Sean McVay, Steve Kerr, Kevin O'Connell, and other successful coaches in various sports.

My approach here is sports-centric. I want to present fitness in the same light as sport.

Fitness should be a joyful, satisfying, and fulfilling experience rather than an intimidating drudgery on your exercise to-do list. It can also be challenging but on your terms.

The bottom line is that if you want your fitness to last a lifetime, you have to move it from the list of things you should do to the list of things you want to do, the things you look forward to. Learn to gamify your fitness activity.

I had the good fortune of having positive, solid coaches in my life, and my success in life's journey is primarily a result of their love and guidance.

It's common to see a tough NFL player in a pregame interview moved to tears when asked about his high school coach. An authentic coach is supportive, nurturing, positive, clear and direct, enthusiastic, and respectful.

A coach builds resiliency by focusing on the future and caring about your long-term success. Positive self-coaching is an integral part of this program.

I've had a variety of titles over the years. Some may sound more prestigious, but none more endearing than the title "coach," which leads to my reason for writing this book—my **WHY.**

For me, particularly at this time of my life, there was only one driving emotion behind my effort to put this project together. It might sound corny, but it's a fact. I spent every day writing this book with one image in mind: the image of one person picking up the book and having it resonate.

While some of these ideas may not work for everyone, I hope you pick up one or two tips and have them click, and as a result, our connection through this book helps you live your best life. That thought, that possibility, gives me deep satisfaction, and the people closest to me know that it is a fact.

No matter my official title for whatever job I was doing at the time—I've always been a supportive coach. I've enjoyed helping people throughout my career and would love to be your coach.

ORIGIN STORY.

> "All advice Is autobiographical. It's one of my theories that when people are giving you advice, they're really just talking about themselves in the past."
>
> —*Steal Like An Artist*, Austin Kleon

Like many, I had a typical, frustrating struggle with exercise adherence. I knew exercise was necessary; it just wasn't happening.

Unknowingly, I had made a subtle but impactful change in my lifestyle that transformed everything. In my late twenties, I left a high school coaching and teaching career to return to grad school to pursue an advanced degree in health behavior, which led to a university teaching position in Health Science.

I thoroughly enjoyed the change, and my days were spent teaching classes in large lecture halls.

The change also had a negative impact on my life that I wasn't expecting. I no longer ran from one end of the football field to the other to work with the linebackers, participate in the team's calisthenic routine, or carry equipment onto the field.

I was now in an office or a classroom—all day. Here, I was teaching about health, and mine was slowly fading.

I could feel it every time I took a flight of stairs. I still enjoyed an occasional ski day in the winter and a little tennis now and then. I'd been a decent high school and college athlete, and I still looked okay clothed, but even that was fading.

Remember, this was in the mid-70s, when the fitness movement, led by Dr. Ken Cooper, was just getting started.

Jogging and/or running was all the rage, so I grabbed my stopwatch, determined to join the new running craze. But I'd been a sprinter in high school and college track and soon discovered I wasn't a distance runner. I wasn't a jogger.

I even had my seven-year-old son, Jeff, ride alongside me on his bike, hoping our conversation would distract from my lack of fun. That didn't help, nor did timing myself each time I ran to see if I could break my personal best. That certainly didn't endear me to this new activity.

The over-the-top competitive instincts that served me well as an athlete became a significant barrier. I was on the proverbial Struggle Bus.

Ironically, at the time, I was teaching an upper-division, graduate-level course focused on behavioral change. The actual course title was "Health Behavior," and it was part of a curriculum that served students training in epidemiology, nursing, and health education.

As part of the class lab project, I had my students choose a behavior they wanted to change.

Applying principles from behavioral psychology, I asked them to write a report that included their successes and frustrations. I also wanted them to give a class presentation at the end of the semester.

On a whim, I announced I would join them in the project, which got a pretty good laugh.

I told them I would work on this little issue I had—exercise. I told the class I knew how to exercise and needed to do it more regularly.

By the way, I should have told them I exercised next to never.

That class project was one of the best learning experiences of my life. It forced me to dig deep and figure out my barriers, roadblocks, and problems.

I created an action plan that incorporated a strategy that was unique at the time but has been embraced by many in the fitness community over the years: the 5-minute rule. We'll review the 5-minute rule in detail and show you how it can be your key to success.

Happily and with gratitude, I can say after all these years that that process keeps giving. It's still with me. It has kept me healthy and sane and gives me satisfaction every day. I have a consistent fitness habit. I'm here to help you find the same joy.

That experience did more than just help me create a fitness habit; it got me deeply interested in the emerging modern fitness industry and was an itch that had to be scratched. So off I went, making a lateral move in a career that maintained a theme—health and fitness.

Along the way, it took the form of fitness club development and management, corporate fitness programming, and a fitness education video series used nationwide for staff training in health and fitness clubs.

The foundation of this book has been created by combining strategies from behavioral science and that class, along with my coaching experiences and involvement in the fitness business and management world—thousands of real-life experiences in real time, working on habits that transform average folks into exercisers.

I also continue to learn daily from people like yourself, working to maintain a healthier life.

FITNESS GETS PERSONAL.

Personal fitness coaching was hardly a thing in 1980. Regular folks didn't have personal trainers come to their homes or work with them in clubs. If you wanted fitness training, you joined a gym, and if you were lucky, maybe you had a friend with a little knowledge to give you a hand.

At this point in my career, I taught strength and conditioning courses at the University of California, San Diego, and was a certified strength and conditioning specialist.

I also worked as a consultant for several fitness equipment manufacturers and companies and developed corporate fitness programs nationwide. Fitness was just starting to emerge in various formats, and I was very busy. I loved it.

One thing led to another, and through this whirlwind of various fitness business activities, I wandered into something fresh. New.

I got into the personal training business by accident. I didn't even know I was doing it.

A friend who owned an exercise equipment company asked me if I would show an important client how to use his new home gym properly. I said sure.

I went over on the given day and guided him through the process. Things went great. He was a pleasant guy and a former college athlete. He had just gotten very busy with life and had a real problem sticking with any kind of exercise routine.

He wanted to learn the proper techniques and how to use the new equipment correctly. As I started to leave, the guy said, "So I'll see you tomorrow at about the same time?"

I started babbling as I usually do when I'm caught off guard, but finally, I realized he was serious and wanted help again early the next morning, so I didn't have an excuse. I wasn't doing anything significant at 6:00 a.m., except maybe sleeping, so I said, "Yeah, I'll help out for a while to make sure you're solid and on track."

He then asked me the awkward question—because I had no idea—"How much do you charge?"

I hesitated; there was no model to follow at that time. As I stood there thinking, he asked if $100 an hour would work. I immediately said yes without flinching. Remember that this was 1983, so a hundred bucks was, well, like, $5,000 in today's money?

Soon, people began asking if I would help them set up a home fitness gym and get started with a program.

Some were well-known people—you could call them celebrities. I even had an NFL Hall of Famer as one of my clients. However, most were just average folks wanting to get in better condition.

But there was one thing that most had in common. They had all exercised before they began training with me, though most had dropped out for one reason or another.

The most common sentiment was, "I never felt better than when I was exercising, and I want to get that feeling back."

They also told me they weren't sure why they'd stopped exercising, except maybe life had just gotten in the way, and before they knew it, they were out of shape.

One thing was sure: They'd struggled with the behavioral side of things, with how to stick with it.

Sure, they wanted some coaching regarding technique; in fact, they were solely focused on their technique. But my focus was also on how I could help them develop a mindset of consistency and help them maintain it, even when I wasn't there with them.

In our follow-up conversations, I learned a lot. I learned what was working for them, why they had slipped up or stopped, and if they had stopped, what helped them to get going again.

So here I was, with my academic training in health behavior, now gaining real-life experience in the world.

I'd work with a client for a few weeks, get them started, and then reconnect a month or two later to find out what had worked and what didn't.

I was interviewed in 1983 about my program, Fitness Success Personal Training, and said, "The problem is that people have too many strict goals.

"They push too hard to accomplish some goal by such a date, and they let their expectations get in their way. And that takes the fun out of it, and eventually, they quit.

"I teach people how to show up, relax, avoid the traps, and enjoy the fitness process.

"Our ultimate secret is to focus on strengthening the exercise habit, knowing that fitness will naturally follow."

That statement is as valid today as it was in 1983.

1.

F.ITNESS A.TTITUDE T.RAINING

How you feel about a particular issue is essential, but you must realize that your attitude doesn't always match your behavior.

For instance, If you fear snakes, I could explain why a non-venomous garter snake is harmless. How important they are to the ecosystem, or how they control pests.

After hearing my explanation, you'd agree intellectually.

But if I dump a bag of those harmless snakes on the table, you'd freak out. I changed your attitude, but clearly, your behavior didn't change.

Still, attitudes are critical in the overall process of behavioral change, and thankfully, they're not set in stone. People can change their outlook or attitude and gradually move toward positive life changes.

HOW DO DOGS SAY EXERCISE?

Attitude is important. So, let's explore something simple as we get started: How do you feel about the word "exercise"? I'm not talking about the concept of exercise; I'm talking about the word, "exercise." Take a moment to say the word and see if you can conjure a feeling. Got it?

Although this may sound trivial, understanding how you feel about that word is sneaky-important; it's a big deal.

I want you for a minute to just feel what that word sounds like at the gut level. If you were being honest, you probably hear that word and think, "It's time to take my medicine. This will not be fun, but it will be worth it."

People who exercise and are successful typically don't hear the word that way. Their brain has developed a different word; in most cases, it's a positive word for satisfaction, enjoyment, or the opportunity to meet a challenge. It's something they want to do and need to do.

The word my brain converts to when I say exercise is "movement." I enjoy getting out and moving.

For most people I work with, achieving that change takes time. Test yourself occasionally as you develop this new habit. How do you feel about the word?

If it's starting to evolve into something that has a more positive connotation, you're getting damn close to being locked in.

Without changing that word and your feelings about it, your chances of success are greatly minimized. Moving from "I've got to" to "I want to" is where the magic happens.

Okay, now the dog part.

What do you think your dog's brain hears when you go toward the door and say, "let's get some exercise"? He hears you say the word "exercise," and his brain interprets that as pure fun and joy—*throw me the ball, throw me the ball, throw me the ball*, and his butt is going 30 miles an hour.

That's sort of how I want you to act when you hear the word "exercise"—just not the butt part.

I KNOW MY PROBLEM; I NEED MOTIVATION.

Any football coach who's ever given what he feels is his best motivational pregame pep talk will tell you that, at best, the motivation from that talk will last about one series of downs.

I was often fooled in the early days of managing my fitness club. People would tell me how motivated they were to start this thing.

And then they were gone.

Surprisingly, the low-key person who came in and accepted that it was a process, moved forward with quiet determination and succeeded at a higher rate. It seemed that there was an inverse correlation.

Motivation has a fast burn rate. Plain and simple, it doesn't last. Motivation and five bucks will get you a cup of coffee at Starbucks.

FOR THE LOVE OF THE GAME.

What's more important than short-term motivation? It's your **why.** I'll explain.

Going back to a football coaching example.

I recently heard a prominent college football coach say in a TV interview that he was always looking for a football player to recruit who played for the right reasons—a player who was not hungry for money, fame, and assorted benefits, but rather for how they feel when they achieve team success—the fun, joy, camaraderie, and fellowship.

The bottom line is: he was looking for players who loved the game. He said he was looking for winning players who had the right **why.**

FINDING YOUR FITNESS WHY.

I want to be healthy and lose some weight, look great, or have a longer health span are some of the responses I typically get when I ask someone about their **why**.

But as you can see, those are pretty general and vague.

While they may hold up during that initial period of high motivation, they tend not to last long-term.

And fear-based **whys** don't have the power. Like, "I don't want to die before my time."

Watch people drive past a horrific accident and move slowly and cautiously for a short distance. Within about a mile, they're all back at full speed and more. You soon feel like you're in a NASCAR race.

Think of it this way: The fundamental core of what inspires you to be active and fit is your **why,** and most likely, when you begin to dig for this, you might touch an emotional cord when you figure out what drives you. This will be more about how you feel than how you think.

It's important not to force this issue. Don't feel you have to come up with an answer right away. Give it time and let it naturally surface.

Often, a person's **reason** can be as simple as enjoying the great feeling, the burst of energy someone gets as they finish their workout. That feeling translates into feeling alive; people want that feeling every day.

I was surprised when I came up with my answer. Initially, I did the same thing everybody did. I gave vague answers: I wanted to live a healthy life, enjoy my recreational activities for as long as possible, and so on. And then I added, "I do it because it's the right thing to do."

That got me curious and caused me to think, what do I mean by, "the right thing to do"? As I pondered that, it hit me. My **why** had a spiritual basis. It was built on a sense of gratitude, deep appreciation, and respect for the gift I have been given . . . my life.

My **why** was focusing on maintaining or caring for that gift with fitness. Consistent exercise.

> **Do you want to know what my favorite part of the game is? The opportunity to play.**
>
> **Mike Singletary,
> Hall of Fame Linebacker**

That attitude, built on gratitude, still gets me out the door. I get to play.

But my **why** is not a conscious thought each day; I rarely think about it. It's just there as a foundation. My daily thought is that I've made a commitment, written my workout into my schedule each day, and want to "do this."

I may not be thrilled when I start my workout, but when I get to a certain point in my routine, most certainly at the finish, I'll say, "I'm really glad I did this."

You may not get that feeling as you begin developing your new fitness routine, but trust me, if you take a reasonable, steady approach, you'll also be glad you did this.

That pleasurable feeling you get as you end your workout is a nice mix of endorphins and self-efficacy thrown in for good measure.

Mastery of a challenging subject is fun. Just be certain you're the one controlling the challenge.

Who doesn't enjoy doing what you set out to do—succeeding?

IT MAY BE TIME!

Sometimes, people successfully change behavior, like sticking with a fitness program, not because of some creative behavioral change strategy but because they've decided that, at long last, they're simply going to make the change.

Many successful behavioral change programs work mainly because participants have heard and considered the pitch several times before. This time, they quietly and calmly determine they've had enough, and it's time to change.

For instance, smokers often quit "cold turkey." They're tired of struggling for years and, out of the blue, decide to quit, commit, and are done.

Whenever I work with somebody to help them restart their fitness program, it's common for them to tell me that they've done this a number of times before and quit.

I'm always patient and explain that it doesn't matter the number of times you've tried and failed; it's the fact that you're continuing to try, and at some point, it's bound to click. I'm always confident it will eventually happen.

Hopefully, this time, something will click—you're due.

My role as a health and fitness hype man is to keep on pitching. I won't give up, and I don't want you to give up.

It's time!

PUT ME IN, COACH, I'M READY!

Your learning readiness, openness to new ideas, and knowledge of how to approach a new project effectively will all greatly improve your chances of success.

The fact that you picked up this book indicates that you're past the contemplation phase and ready to move on to the most crucial phase—action!

No matter what you might be targeting, whether it's becoming more consistent with your current fitness program or going for a fresh restart, being ready to learn is key.

In the book *Tiny Habits,* author BJ Fogg, PhD, presents two maxims of behavior change. Maxim #1: "Help people do what they already want to do." Maxim #2: "Help people feel successful."

That reminds me of one of my favorite stories about readiness.

Paratroopers during the Second World War were subjected to an accelerated training program. There wasn't much time to spare to get them up to speed and ready.

Training started with the basics: These are the planes we'll be jumping from. This is the theory of aerodynamics and how your chutes function. Here are the things you need to remember... on and on.

As they moved into a large room for instruction, the instructor, standing at a large table in the front, said, "This is my parachute, and there's one just like it in front of you. I will go step by step, teaching you how to fold and pack your parachute." He then made the statement that got their attention and guaranteed their learning readiness was at an all-time high.

He said, "Gentlemen, when we're finished with this exercise, we'll take the parachute you just folded and packed and go to the aircraft out on the tarmac, and you'll be taking your first jump with that chute. Do I have your attention?"

I don't need that kind of attention, but I hope you're ready to look at this issue from a slightly different perspective and become the consistent exerciser you've always wanted to be.

AWARENESS IS A GAME CHANGER.

Awareness, combined with self-awareness, is the ability to observe what is happening around you and your environment. It also includes looking inward and examining your attitudes, feelings, behaviors, and thoughts. That set of skills is vital to your fitness success.

Dr Judson Brewer, M.D., states: "Awareness itself may be enough to change behavior."

So take some time and think back to your last restart, or for that matter, all of the times you've tried to establish your fitness routine. In that process, you can cultivate an awareness of what went right and what went wrong. Your mindset should be one of curiosity.

Did I create stress in my routine because I was unrealistic? Did I push myself to lose 10 pounds by June 1? Did I commit myself to going to the gym four days a week after work, no matter what?

Did I try the "sweat is the sign of weakness, leaving your body" gonzo approach? Was I trying to connect with my inner beast, only to realize I wasn't David Goggins?

Or did I label myself hopeless and quit simply because I'd missed a few workouts? I felt great; and maybe if I had thought I didn't have to be perfect, I could have kept going.

The key is to reflect and study yourself to gain insight. Awareness is not some airy-fairy thing; it's nothing more than paying attention and being curious.

Now, remember we're going to bring much more to the table than just awareness, but it's worth your time to be introspective. It's a vital first step, and as you perfect your awareness skills, you'll start getting your fit back.

TRUST THE PROCESS—RELAX YOUR GRIP.

> Relax and stay in the process; shape happens!
>
> —Sean Gale

Desperation coupled with a strong desire for the perfect outcome is, in most cases, a recipe for disaster. The secret is to have a plan, a sequence of steps that keep you locked into the process of getting fit.

Your plan will start with baby steps and have a built-in adjustment mechanism that gets you back on track when things go a little off. Things are bound to go off track from time to time.

Golfers know things start going sideways when they grip the club too tightly. A relaxed grip leads to a smoother, more successful performance. The same deal applies to fitness: relax and keep your effort under control; consistency over time is the winning formula.

Remember: You can't get in shape today but can keep the ball rolling down the field. With small steps every day, shape happens.

TRUST THE PROCESS—STAY IN THE MOMENT.

Coaches know that getting ahead of yourself in any game creates significant problems.

Possibly the most cliche phrase in football is, "one play at a time."

A new phrase or cliche has come into vogue recently, and I like it better. And that phrase is, "next play."

We can't change the previous play or workout. You may have had a great walk or missed a workout.

But that's history, and we can't do anything about it. All we can do is step up in the present and perform—perform our fundamentals and run the play we have.

Modern coaches realize that winning isn't something they can control. All they can do is run each play to the best of their ability, feel good about their effort and execution when it's over, and let the score take care of itself.

They know one thing for sure: stressing over the outcome and focusing on the score decreases the likelihood that they will win the game.

How does this pertain to you and your fitness program? Simply put, the key to your consistent fitness program will be showing up at the walking path, the trailhead, or the gym and doing the next set or striding down the trail.

Stop demanding that you grind out a spectacular session and produce a personal best that day.

Go ahead and challenge yourself if you'd like, but no matter what, keep your focus on chipping away. Small, imperceptible gains lead to big improvements and ongoing success.

BUT HOW WILL I KNOW IF I'M SUCCEEDING?

How will you know if you're winning the game?

Again, you need to tap into your new and developing awareness skills.

You've worked out for the past six weeks and realize you're taking a flight of stairs and you're not out of breath, your clothes don't feel tight, and you're falling to sleep much easier. You're pooping on the regular again.

You're slowly becoming fit-*ish,* aware of the subtle little wins, the rewards.

Many people don't see the rewards immediately, particularly at the beginning of their program. This is often because they don't know where to look.

One afternoon, I wandered around my fitness club, acting like a maitre d' in a good restaurant.

The role of a maitre d' is to touch base with folks and see how you can help them get the most out of their experience.

I touched base with my members to see how things were going.

As I was circulating in my gym, having conversations with various people about how things were going for them and their programs, I had an experience that opened my eyes to this whole awareness issue.

One of my members was walking toward the door and just gave me a nod and a smile, and I said, "Hey, how's everything going?" He responded, "Pretty good, but I'm just not losing the weight I'd hoped. I wanted to get down to like 175."

His comment caught me off guard; he'd been conscientious about his training and was making quite an improvement.

So, I reminded him of something I discuss with everyone when they start a strength training program.

I explained that getting stronger builds lean body mass and loses body fat. Don't be surprised when you step on the scale to find that you may be heavier.

Just remember you're losing body fat, gaining some muscle, and getting healthier.

He responded, "But I sure hope I can get to 175."

I have no idea where that number came from, but in my experience, everybody has this number, this "ideal" weight thing.

My philosophy has always been, let's get in shape and see the number. Just relax and keep working out. You'll look and feel better; who cares what the number is?

To demonstrate that knowledge or intelligence had nothing to do with this member's attitude—his emotional connection to some arbitrary number—consider this: the guy in question was a physician.

As we talked, I felt disappointed that I hadn't gotten through to this guy, and I could see his disappointment.

Then I started thinking, scanning, and wondering what I could say to keep his spirits up.

And then I saw it. I looked at his belt buckle, and there was a noticeable two or three notches from its previous settings. And I said, "Eric, how long have those marks been on your belt?"

I said, "Eric, that's happening because you're losing body fat." He thought for a second and said, "Yeah, you're right."

That event was so beneficial to my growth as a fitness guy. It made me aware of how important it is to teach people to be aware of a wide range of subtle, positive changes that go on during the fitness process.

Ultimately, this awareness is tied to the reward system of the "habit loop" and can be the difference between success and failure.

THE BEST ABILITY IS ADAPTABILITY.

"Everybody has a plan until they get punched in the mouth."

—Mike Tyson

Coaches often say that an athlete's best ability is his availability.

If an athlete is injured and can't play, no matter the talent level, he can't help the team in the training room.

Another very important ability, particularly in maintaining consistency in your fitness program, is the concept of adaptability.

My college football coach, John Scolinos, often mentioned that the ability to adapt to changing conditions during a football play separates the good defensive player from the great defensive player.

Anyone can make the play when everything's going right, but the great ones adapt and adjust. The critical skill is reading on the move, assessing things, and making the proper adjustments.

Adaptability is also vital for anyone working to maintain a fitness program.

Most of the time, people do a good job when things are going smoothly—everything's perfect, and there are no changes in schedule.

But for almost everyone; there are times when life gets in the way of our fitness routine.

You just got a new promotion, are recovering from a serious injury, have moved, or are in a new relationship.

The important thing is to have a simple foundation that you can return to when circumstances change.

A foundational structure is the key to getting your program back on track.

None other than fitness legend Arnold Schwarzenegger talks about enjoying the challenge of pushing yourself to your limits but knowing that the key to longevity in your fitness program is adaptability.

WHEN DO YOU BECOME FIT?

World ski champion Mikaela Shiffrin is a skier. Your friend Jordon just skied a few times this season and, in reality, is a hack. But he probably calls himself a skier. He looks forward to skiing and any opportunity to improve his game. After all, he's a skier.

Mat Fraser, CrossFit champion, is fit and beyond. In comparison, you've just restarted your fitness program and are not nearly as fit as you'd like.

Are you a fitness person? My answer would be yes. You're in the fitness process. Mat and you both have the same objective: getting fitter. Nobody ever truly gets there; it's a process.

Someone who sees themselves as a slacker and is trying to get fit is setting themselves up for failure. However, someone who sees themselves as fit can begin to make decisions throughout their life that a fit person would make.

Going for a walk when there's a break in your day is what a fit person does. Making a better food choice aligns with how you see yourself—as a fit person.

I know it may feel odd. It's different, and you're getting the hang of a new routine, but please, as soon as possible, try to begin thinking of yourself proudly as a fit person.

In his excellent book *Atomic Habits*, James Clear states that true behavior change is identity change. "Improvements are only temporary until they become part of who you are."

KEEP IT SIMPLE.

As you reset and start your program again, try to avoid getting lost in information overload.

For most, the struggle is not a lack of information but the lack of simply doing the simple—emphasis on *doing*.

Now, let me clarify: I'm not talking about individuals involved in the competitive aspects of fitness and sport. They're looking for any edge to optimize training, and their training protocols can be pretty complex.

But getting restarted is straightforward for most people who use fitness simply to feel better, have more energy, and get more out of life.

I suggest a check-up from your primary care physician who can give you the go-ahead for a basic exercise program. Once that's done, you can start your Almost Consistent Fitness action plan. It doesn't get any simpler than that.

> **EXERCISE IS MEDICINE**
>
> "The first thing people notice is, I feel better, I have more energy, I sleep better... The curve is very steep in terms of the benefits, doing just a little bit gives tremendous benefits. So I try to focus on those smaller pieces instead of feeling like you have to join a gym and you have to do all this. Just go out and walk."
>
> An NBC interview with Dr Robert Sallis M.D., past president of the American College of Sports Medicine and practicing physician who inspired the "Exercise is Medicine" campaign.

IS A SIMPLE, RELATIVELY EASY FITNESS ROUTINE EFFECTIVE?

Dr. Peter Attia, M.D., physician and author explains that even the most basic exercise provides tremendous benefits. He refers to this easier form of exercise as low-hanging fruit.

There is no question that training for advanced levels of fitness has significant benefits, but a substantial percentage of those benefits are gained from simple exercise, often referred to as Zone 2 training.

We'll cover the basics of putting together a good walking program, including how to buy the right shoe and the left one. I will present a tip or two about posture, the basics of the talk test, and how to determine if you're in Zone 2 and getting a training effect.

Dr. Michael Joyner, M.D. of the Mayo Clinic, also a competitive runner, offers what I think is the perfect strategy for people who want to start exercising:

1. Find something to do that is sustainable and do it every day.
2. Do 30 minutes of activity daily that you can break down into 10-minute bouts.
3. Reduce the sedentary time in your life whenever you can, such as parking further away in parking lots.

The bottom line is that your daily exercise session, as well as spontaneous additional activity throughout the day, create a synergy that's vital in your quest of becoming more fit. Think of building awareness around these two important aspects of your training. I refer to it as using your motion detector.

> **Time is the coin of your life. It is the only coin you have, and only you can determine how it will be spent. Be careful lest you let other people spend it for you.**
>
> —Carl Sandberg

2.

SELF-SABOTAGE, BARRIERS, AND TRAPS.

So you have this great attitude. You're looking forward to fitness becoming a great addition to your life. You've been fit in the past and want to get fit again. You know it's the right thing to do, but you're not doing it...yet!

And it's beginning to eat at you, making you uncomfortable—a little self-loathing starts to creep in.

Your brain generates a B.S. story: "I'm pretty busy this week; let's wait until the first of the month."

Ah, the old procrastination trick.

This is self-sabotage in full bloom. You're arguing with yourself, and your subconscious is lobbying for the easy way out, desperate to feel better about itself. It's winning the argument, but in the end, you lose.

In the 1950s, psychologist Leon Festinger developed the term *cognitive dissonance* for this behavior. In short, when your attitude conflicts with your behavior, you feel discomfort and want to protect your ego.

The easy way out of this discomfort is to devise a reason. The perfect reason!

We're all great at lying to ourselves to eliminate the discomfort, and it's effective. However, you're still stuck with the problem.

For instance, someone could have a smoking habit and understand the serious health consequences down the road. That makes them uncomfortable and creates dissonance.

Then, the smoker devises the perfect rationalization: "You don't live forever." Or, "I saw a 90-year-old guy who smoked his whole life, and he was doing push-ups on YouTube."

Another example is someone who doesn't wear a seatbelt. They're quick to tell you the story of someone who was thrown from a crash which saved their life because the car burst into flames.

You might explain that the statistical probabilities of that are off the charts. The sharpies in Las Vegas call that a moonshot, but it doesn't matter; it just makes them feel better about their behavior.

When someone tells you they don't have time for exercise, but you are aware of their daily screen time, you know that excuse simply doesn't wash. But it does make them feel better.

You could throw the B.S. Challenge Flag, but you'd soon realize they would devise a better excuse on the spot. The excuse-generating machine keeps on giving.

When our behavior doesn't match our attitude, we have two choices: We can change our attitude about the behavior, or better yet, we can change our behavior.

One solution to this dilemma is to be aware. I've already discussed awareness, which comes into play when you hear yourself making excuses for not doing something.

Ask yourself: What am I getting out of this? Why don't I have time? Can I make this task easier?

How can I reduce the friction and smooth my way into an exercise habit? Could I find a way around boredom? There has to be a way to make this more fun.

The ultimate trick is to make exercise an easier option than making up some weak ass excuse. Okay, it may not be easier, but it could be close.

And you get the satisfaction of not lying to yourself.

To help find a solution, you can learn a lot by simply being curious. What's holding me back? Examine your excuses.

I know that when I was floundering around and finding it difficult to exercise, my excuses were that it was no fun and, on top of that, boring.

Behind those excuses are the real reasons. Number one, I didn't find it fun because I used my old 'no pain, no gain' strategy. That strategy worked in my athletic background but didn't work in establishing an exercise routine, so it wasn't fun.

Number two, it was boring because I was pushing myself through a lot of pain and discomfort, and it's incredible how slowly time moves when you're in pain.

My fix: The ultimate solution to my problem revolved around addressing those issues. I needed to find a mechanism that reduced the pressure of achieving a certain amount by a specific date and simply gain control of my intensity.

I had to learn that I wouldn't get in shape the day I started exercising—it's a process that requires small, consistent steps in order to see results.

Oh yeah, I almost forgot. For good measure, I offered the excuse that I didn't have time. This was total B.S. I was busy, but I had time.

Ultimately, self-awareness can give you essential insights into what's going on, what roadblocks keep you from success, and how you might navigate them. This can make all the difference between success and defeat.

Here are a few common roadblocks, barriers, and traps to a consistent fitness program.

I DON'T HAVE TIME.

> "I don't have time to exercise because... I don't want to."
>
> —Jim Gaffigan

You want to get in shape, but you don't have the time.

Who doesn't have a problem with priorities in our day-to-day life? Nobody.

Warren Buffett offers an excellent time management suggestion when he asks his audience to list and rank their priorities in life from 1 to 25. Now, focus on the first five and do your best to avoid the remaining 20.

If taking care of yourself with a consistent fitness routine is not high on that list, you need a new list.

Prioritize and schedule.

There are several ways to schedule.

You can schedule well in advance, maybe a week ahead, or you may need an adaptable daily schedule strategy in which you commit to working your exercise in sometime before the end of your day. You look for gaps or opportunities and make them happen.

As you begin your airline flight, the announcement says it best: If there's an emergency, put your oxygen mask on first and then help your kids. If you pass out, you can't help others. A daily fitness break is your oxygen mask.

A great way to solve the time issue for many is bundling. For instance, pick a daily activity, such as watching television. The solution for many is to combine watching TV with exercise. It's simple: put a bike, treadmill, or elliptical in front of the TV and exercise while watching your favorite show.

I occasionally put a favorite football game on delay and then walk on my treadmill for the whole game. I can fast-forward through the commercials, and obviously, I have a comfortable pace, but I do get in a good exercise session doing something I enjoy: watching a good football game.

My favorite bundling strategy is listening to podcasts while taking a walk. The walk might be an opportunistic 15 minutes in the morning or a planned 45 minutes at the end of the work day.

I enjoy a variety of podcasts. I just have one rule: I can only listen to podcasts while walking. So, I look forward to my walk and my podcast.

I was driving through town one day recently and saw a group of parents in a park, waiting for their kids to finish a sports practice.

Off to the side of the group, I saw an athletic young woman doing lunges. I did a double-take, realizing it was my daughter-in-law Ashley, who was also waiting to pick up their three kids after the practice. There she was, involved in the classic multitasking mode, grabbing an opportunity during her very busy day to get a portion of her exercise routine done.

Ashley is a working mom with a demanding schedule. She's a physician who works long hours, often on call at the hospital late into the night. Yet she finds a way to maintain her fitness activities through creative scheduling and a quiet determination to get it done.

Incredibly busy people who prioritize can be successful in their exercise habits. Surprisingly, many of these types view exercise as not a time-waster but an energy source.

Some people who struggle with exercise think that people who are consistent and able to find the time for exercise are different. It's not hard for them; they have a natural gift or extra time on their hands. Wrong. I had to figure out where to fit my exercise into my schedule—today.

I don't know how many times someone has told me about their struggles, and said that I probably couldn't identify with them because exercise was undoubtedly easy for me, implying that it's a genetic gift to be fit.

Whenever somebody makes that comment, I realize how annoyed successful athletes get when folks assume they've won the genetic lottery. Those athletes always know of somebody better than them when they began the process but failed to put in the time or effort.

There's no question that they have a genetic advantage, but their success is based on their work ethic: making the time, showing up, and always striving to improve themselves. They crush it with their attitude. They're consistent.

We all have that same opportunity to maximize the gifts we've been given.

Finding time simply means valuing or caring enough to choose exercise over something else.

> When you say one of these days, you mean never.
>
> —Anonymous

Julie was a member of my fitness club. She was a single mom who was a teacher and also worked part-time to help meet her family's needs.

The fitness club opened every day at 6:00 a.m. I was talking to Julie and just touching base to see how everything was going in her program, and she asked me if I could open at 5:00 a.m.

She had difficulty getting everything into her day; a 5:00 a.m. start would be perfect.

I gave her my business reasons for not opening at 5:00 a.m.: one, I didn't believe we would have any customers other than herself, and the other, it was hard enough finding somebody reliable who could open at 6:00 a.m., and 5:00 a.m. would probably be impossible.

Then she came up with a suggestion. She told me she was willing to be trained as a staff member and already had a CPR certificate.

Could she open the gym each morning at 5:00? She said she would gladly do it for free.

Done.

Once we opened at 5:00, a surprising number of members began showing up at the earlier hour, and I quickly made her a paid staff member.

Being flexible and resourceful is crucial to solving time issues.

By the way, I've had an easier time helping people develop fitness habits who have incredibly busy schedules than those who have more free time.

It's the thing: if you want something done, give it to a busy person.

IT'S BORING.

> Exercise is not boring; you're boring.
>
> —Dr. George Sheehan

Pleasant distractions are the key to eliminating boredom.

I learned this years ago when fitness clubs didn't have computerized, gamified cardio equipment. Our only cardio equipment was exercise bikes with a weighted flywheel, a friction strap, and a manual timer. There were no spin classes; you were alone with your thoughts. Now, that could get boring!

We now have a better solution—interactive consoles, AirPods, podcasts, or music.

Learning to relax and finding a comfortable level of exertion while walking and listening to your favorite podcast can help you overcome boredom. You can even learn a foreign language or listen to a book while you walk.

So, if you're on a fitness walk, you can opt for some onboard entertainment or unplug from the noise and enjoy the flow of creativity and the sounds of nature.

A daily splash of natural light delivers vitamin D and helps regulate your sleep cycles. Turns out that exposure to nature's flora and fauna is good for you.

Either strategy is a winner.

HOW CAN PEOPLE SAY THIS IS FUN?

> "Takin' on a challenge is a lot like riding a horse. If you're comfortable while you're doing it, you're probably doin' it wrong."
>
> —Ted Lasso

Lots of activities can be awkward and uncomfortable when you begin, but they can become spectacular given time. And no, I'm not talking about *that* activity; I'm trying to keep this book G-rated.

A perfect example of a person discovering whether they like something or not was my experience—and struggle—learning to ski. Everyone told me skiing was a blast.

However, the first few times I tried it, I hated it.

If you've ever skied, you might relate.

I was in my mid-20s, and a cousin of mine, a ski instructor, took me to the hill one Saturday to try it. The boots were painfully uncomfortable, my balance was non-existent, and for a reasonably competent athlete, I was flopping around and having zero fun...

I went for my second ski experience a week later just to see if it sucked as bad as I thought it did.

It still sucked, but not quite as bad. So now I was curious.

I went for a third visit to the slopes, and I still didn't have it all together, but my comfort level was going up. I began to glimpse the possibility of being able to navigate the hill.

I soon became an obsessed skier; couldn't get enough.

This is precisely what the fitness journey is like for lots of people.

It can be very misleading to someone who's just getting started. The bubbly and charismatic group fitness instructor shouting, "Let's have fun today!" may cause you to think, "What am I missing?"

You're doing all the right things but failing in the fun department.

The most successful long-term exercisers learn to get enjoyment over time and at various levels.

Some learn to enjoy meeting a physical challenge or accomplishment, like walking further or lifting more, achieving a personal best, or running a marathon in under 3 hours—the satisfaction of doing hard things.

They may also have developed a social bond with friends and enjoy getting together for the same activity: a sweat-producing yoga class, a brisk walk with a friend, or a group bike ride.

But no one who's a consistent exerciser fails to get a good feeling from each exercise session. It may be tough at the start of your routine, but once you get a rhythm and that endorphin boost kicks in, you feel good. And almost every time, you end up feeling, "I'm glad I did that."

So, having fun is a learned process, and I'm still working on it, but I usually manage to pull it off...mostly.

The best approach is to lower your fun expectations, take a baby-step approach to physical effort, and be patient.

Keep in mind that the most crucial emotion is that you look forward to doing it again.

I can always sense when somebody is locked into the habit. They're unhappy when they miss a fitness walk.

They've taken exercise to the habit level and changed their thought process from, *I have to*, to *I want to*.

ALL-OR-NOTHING—
STAY OUT OF THE PAIN CAVE!

> "Intensity makes a lot of noise, but if you have the real dog in you, you have consistency. Consistency always wins."
>
> —RPM

The all-or-nothing mindset will sabotage even the most determined exerciser.

Unbridled intensity and a dash of perfectionism are extremely common roadblocks to fitness success. Athletes refer to this level of intensity as the pain cave. Don't go in there!

The famous Vince Lombardi quote, "Fatigue makes cowards of us all," could easily be modified to say, "Fatigue and pain lead to procrastination—which makes cowards of us all."

Until I solved the all-or-nothing aspect of my fitness program, I was destined to be an inconsistent on-and-off exerciser.

> Something is better than nothing if it's consistent.
>
> —Dr. Ken Cooper

Dr. Ken Cooper said it best: "Taking fitness beyond a certain point is often done for reasons other than fitness." Marathons or CrossFit competitions are great at testing your fitness limits and can get you pretty deep into the pain cave, but they go well beyond most people's needs for a basic fitness routine.

Our job here is to develop the habit of consistent, moderate exercise.

In high-performance competitive athletics, it's understandable that athletes must push themselves close to the edge. However, even they need the right level of intensity to produce the results.

An all-or-nothing mindset can lead to overtraining, negative outcomes, and, ultimately, burnout.

Whether you're an athlete in training or starting a basic fitness program, the all-or-nothing mindset is the enemy. At the root of that mindset is a desire to get the best possible results—now!

Sports psychology suggests a solution to this problem. Stop focusing on outcomes and results. Stick with a well-designed, consistent training plan. Stop looking ahead. Stay patient and chip away, chop by chop.

They refer to this as the "process." The one-play-at-a-time mentality: you're not looking ahead.

You don't have the baggage of high expectations for the perfect long-term outcome; you just show up, execute your fundamentals, and come back tomorrow and do the same thing.

In baseball, there's a superstition. Nobody talks to the pitcher who is in the process of throwing a no-hitter. The dugout is quiet. They don't want him to focus on the outcome. They want him to keep throwing the ball and not overthink the situation.

The same mindset is perfect for you as you start or restart your fitness program. Don't look forward. Just keep showing up, and the results will come.

The paradox in my fitness journey was that I started to get fit when I gave up perfectionism, the need for maximum effort in every workout, and unrealistic expectations.

Success in the long-term is all about enjoying success in the moment. And that feeds success tomorrow.

STRENGTH TRAINING.

Although I won't discuss specific techniques and strategies in this book, I'd like to mention strength training. It should be an integral part of any comprehensive fitness program.

However, consider adding strength training after firmly establishing your daily walking habit. Trying to make a multitude of changes at the same time is typically not very effective.

> "I don't mean to be sacrilegious, but I truly believe that if Jesus returned to Earth during these times, he'd lift weights."
>
> Red Lerille, a Former Mr. America,
> Speaking at a Fitness Industry Conference

In the early days of the modern fitness movement, strength training was not a priority. However, research scientists like Dr. William Evans changed that thinking. His research, along with others, demonstrated how vital strength training was to people's quality of life.

Arthur Jones, an entrepreneur who developed the Nautilus training system, began a wave of interest in strength training, and today, it's hotter than hot.

And even though strength training is popular with facilities on almost every corner, gym environments can feel uncomfortable when you first show up—whether using cardio equipment, joining a group class, or using strength training equipment.

One of the best things you can do if you feel uncomfortable in a gym setting is to turn down the volume when comparing yourself to others.

And if you're concerned that the super fit are making judgments about your lack of fitness, know that typically, they really aren't. At least not the ones who are truly fit.

Most have traveled a similar road and give you nothing but respect.

To them, the important thing is that you're going about it the right way. You're learning the fundamentals, how to use the equipment, and basic etiquette.

By the way, there's an essential piece of etiquette that people don't typically tell you but is a good thing to know: don't stand in a bodybuilder's sight line to a mirror.

I say that half joking, but it illustrates that the focus is not on you.

Beyond feeling self-conscious, there are other issues to deal with.

There's equipment you may not be familiar with, or maybe the layout's different. Ask for an orientation. Almost every gym I've ever been to will have somebody more than happy to give you a hand getting started.

And one last thing: regarding strength training at the gym, your routine does not need to be a long, drawn out ordeal.

It's unfortunate, but I often see beginners wandering around a fitness facility clutching their water bottles, struggling on an exercise machine with not-so-great form, and resting between sets much longer than necessary.

Most people who want a basic strength training program can achieve success in just 30 to 60 minutes, three times a week. You can extend your sessions in the future if strength training becomes more of a priority.

> An up-tempo training strategy with relatively short rest intervals works well from a physiological and behavioral standpoint. You will get stronger, and you'll be a lot happier doing it.
>
> A qualified personal trainer can teach you how to make the most of your time and how to do the exercises properly.

MY WORKOUT PARTNER QUIT.

The conventional wisdom is to tell folks that working out or walking with a friend is a great way to stick to their fitness program. Well, I would give that suggestion a definite "maybe."

The strategy of training with a friend may get you started, but as soon as possible, try to think of yourself as training independently—alongside a friend. Because if your friend is like a lot of friends, you'll soon be training solo.

I think it's pretty obvious, but if you're codependent with a walking partner and one of you quits, there's a high likelihood that the other one will quit, too. I saw it time and time again in my fitness clubs.

Workout partners aren't the only issue in this regard. Some people fall in love with a particular fitness club, then move and can't get started again. If they go to a group exercise class and lock in on a favorite teacher, but then the teacher leaves, they leave too.

I'm like the Farmers Insurance guy; I've seen it all.

If you plan to make exercise a lifetime habit, and I hope that's your choice, the best strategy is learning how to enjoy your own company. That's the person you can rely on throughout the lifetime process.

Enjoy the friends you train with and the classes you join. But most importantly, learn to cherish the time you spend with yourself.

INJURED RESERVE (I.R.)

I'm a fitness coach, not a physician. As mentioned, I encourage everyone who starts or restarts their fitness program to touch base with their primary care physician.

Undoubtedly, the highest risk behavior is sitting on the couch and doing nothing. Sedentary behavior is even riskier than smoking, but if you haven't had a checkup in a while, I encourage you to do so.

Active people will invariably deal with injury and also get hurt.

What's the difference, you say? When an athlete is hurt, that typically refers to soreness or general muscle discomfort from pushing themselves a bit while training or practicing.

However, when someone is injured, it's more severe and potentially damaging if they continue to train. It's not something you can work through. It must be taken seriously and should typically be examined by a physical therapist or a physician.

The distinction between those two things is sometimes difficult to make. If you have experience and realize this is just soreness from an exercise you recently modified, that's one thing. But if it's something new on the radar, and certainly if it's getting worse, it's time to get some guidance.

Whenever I've been injured in my routine, it's typically caused by overuse. If I back off and it still does not get better, I get it checked out.

When I'm hurting, I typically try to find a work-around.

For example, suppose I have a foot or toe problem that acts up when I take a full stride in my walk. In that case, I might opt for a few days on the elliptical machine, hopefully eliminating the pain while still allowing me to maintain my cardiovascular conditioning.

Whatever you do, don't pound on an injury to the point that you damage yourself and put your long-term mobility at risk. Put yourself on I.R., then get it checked out.

3.

THINK HABITS.

> "The chains of habit are too weak to be felt until they are too strong to be broken."
>
> —Samuel Johnson

For a long time, the conventional wisdom in fitness training was, "Get people fit as soon as possible so you can show them results. Sure, be gradual and steady with the programming, but always remember it's vital to show them results, or they won't stick with it."

My experience has been different. Over the years, I've interviewed thousands of people trying to restart their exercise programs, and it's amazing how many of them look back at their previous programs and say they loved the results they got. Still, for one reason or another, they quit. They didn't quit because they didn't get results. What's going on?

The answer is simple. Remove the focus from results and expectations and establish an easy, effective habit based on feeling better and having more energy—in the present moment.

Take pride in your commitment to something that you know will benefit you. Take pride in doing something that others might find difficult. Love your effort.

Have no fear; results will happen over time, but the secret to keeping those results long-term is simple: you need to develop a consistent exercise habit, or you'll always be locked into an on-again/off-again exercise pattern.

Build your habit with the help of our Habit Streak Tracker.

The habit of consistent exercise is the solution.

THE HABIT LOOP.

> "Even if you're on the right track, you will get run over if you just sit there."
>
> —Will Rogers

Webster defines a habit as "a usual way of behaving or a tendency that someone has settled into." Consistency begets consistency.

In his exceptional book *Atomic Habits*, James Clear refers to a four-step model, commonly known as a "habit loop": cue, craving, response, and reward.

James Clear developed a set of rules called the "laws of behavior change."

1. It should be obvious.
2. It should be attractive.
3. It should be manageable.
4. It should be satisfying.

Another way of framing this is: awareness, joyful anticipation, and a task so easy you can't refuse, followed by a reward.

This is the perfect strategy for building lasting habits.

The habit most often used to explain the "habit loop" is brushing your teeth.

You wake up groggy, look in the mirror, and then glance down and see your toothbrush. You automatically pick up your toothbrush, put some toothpaste on it, and brush your teeth. You then rinse out your mouth and feel the refreshing, cool taste of fresh breath.

In an exercise habit, the cue might be waking up and seeing your workout gear placed in an obvious location. You put it on and head out the door for your morning walk.

Once you get a rhythm in your stride, you enjoy the action of your morning walk.

You feel invigorated as you complete your walk, and the reward of a tasty, protein-rich strawberry smoothie awaits.

And you give yourself another reward. You make a mark in your "Fitness Success Tracker," which feels great. You kept your fitness streak alive another day—bonus plus bonus.

Everybody's day is different, and your cue may be different too.

For instance, a scheduled reminder pops up on your phone. You choose an activity, such as 30 minutes on an exercise bike at the gym, and your reward may be an ice-cold bottle of flavored water and the podcast you listen to.

Personally, the reward that is the most powerful and gives me an incredible amount of satisfaction—though don't get me wrong—I love a good smoothie—is the pride I take in my effort.

I showed up, and the average guy is still in bed! Good job.

Prominent neuroscientist Andrew Huberman says pride and effort have a neurological basis. You produce dopamine, and the subsequent rush helps you strengthen the habit. I'm buying it.

How do you know when your exercise habit is solid?

The rule of thumb I use is simply this: You know you have a solid habit—you're locked in—if you were forced to skip the scheduled exercise session and miss it. You miss the good feelings you get from your workout. You're disappointed, and you look forward to getting back on the horse tomorrow.

That's the moment you know you have a secure habit.

The more you do the routine/ habit, the more solid it becomes. My 8-year-old granddaughter Lula asked me the other day what I was writing about, and I explained the "habit loop" concept and how you know a habit is solid.

She said, "Oh, you mean on autopilot." Nailed it.

IT'S NOT SO HARD—JUST SLIDE IN.

"The secret of getting ahead is getting started."

—Mark Twain

Social scientist Dr. Wendy Wood discusses another exciting way to develop a solid habit: understanding friction. By recognizing the barriers and forces around you, and reducing that friction, you can enhance your ability to form lasting habits.

Remove the barriers. Make it so easy to do something, that it's impossible or nearly impossible to say no.

The classic car sales line is, "What's it going to take to put you in a car today?" In other words, what barriers do I need to remove to get you to buy a car today?

Lower payments, more significant discounts, a different color, or whatever. That's how the salesman begins to figure out where you have resistance—so he can then remove those barriers.

If he can knock those barriers down, he'll be able to slide you smoothly and effortlessly into that new car today.

Another classic example is the buffet. The food is abundant and right there. You don't have to ask for it; just take a few steps and fill your plate again. That's almost zero friction.

And who hasn't had the experience of signing up for a subscription online with almost zero friction or barriers to entry? Press a button, and your monthly subscription will be charged to your card. So, the company has removed all the friction and let you in.

Okay, now try to stop that subscription. Their strategy is simple: create friction. There are many steps and loops; of course, they hope you give up. They keep you in the deal unless you're persistent.

Dr Wood discusses a company's experiment to see if it can get its employees to use the stairs instead of the elevator.

The health benefits of using the stairs are apparent, so the company put up signs asking people to use the stairs instead of the elevator, saying it is healthier. However, the use of the stairs remained the same.

Then, the company did something interesting: they created a delay in the opening of the elevator doors, so people had to wait a short period before getting on the elevator.

After making this relatively simple change, a delay in opening the doors, people began using the stairs.

In effect, the stairs were the easier option. "The hell with it. I'll use the stairs."

She points out that an interesting aspect of the study was when the doors were back to normal speed, the people who started using the stairs kept using them.

So, with all that in mind, your objective should be to do whatever it takes to make things easier.

For instance, take the pressure off yourself. Don't be intimidated by a one-hour gut-wrenching, sweat-producing workout. Think of it as showing up for a short, easy session; if you want to do more, you can.

Or, to use the bundling concept, make some calls while walking on the treadmill for 20 minutes.

By the way, you can get rid of a bad habit by reversing the concept of friction.

I love chips—let me repeat that—I *love* chips. And I have no discipline or willpower to deal with them. But I have a solution, and it's obvious and simple: I don't buy chips!

There are still chips somewhere, like the grocery store, but I'm home. I'm kicked back and comfortable, and I won't drive to the store to get some. It would be too much hassle and friction.

4.

THINK PROCESS, NOT GOALS.

> **Faith and hope are wonderful things, but I do not like them to necessarily be strategies.**
>
> Kevin O'Connell,
> NFL Head Coach

THE PROCESS—TRUST IT!

John Wooden was a personal hero.

The legendary UCLA basketball coach was asked at a presser if he had a goal of a 20-win season. He smiled and said, "We'll practice our fundamentals, and the wins will take care of themselves."

That's the process before it was called—the process.

Bill Walsh, the San Francisco 49ers' Super Bowl-winning coach, followed Coach Wooden's lead and was one of the first to introduce the concept of the process.

When asked about his goals for the season, he quickly deflected the question and said he would focus on what made his team better and practice each day to improve.

His focus was not on winning the Super Bowl, some far-off and uncontrollable result, but on getting better every day—the process.

That concept evolved and was passed on to contemporary NFL coaches like Sean McVay and Kevin McConnell, who continue to train their teams in incremental improvement every day.

You take the concept into the game and focus on the next play, the next shot. You control the things you can control.

This habit thing is all about a series of small, consistent wins over time that can make a huge difference.

Brushing your teeth one time is worthless, but a lifetime of brushing daily gives you optimal dental health. Small, consistent wins produce big-time results.

Business types have a saying that any time you can make a profit on a business deal, be happy to make the profit, no matter the size, and move on. A series of these small profit opportunities ultimately lead to wealth.

GOALS VS. SYSTEMS.

Success comes from a system or process. It's not willpower, luck, motivation, goals, or a game face.

In my experience working with folks over the years, I realized that, for the most part, people who are successful in their program and those who drop out have one thing in common: they have goals.

We could nitpick about the quality of their goals or their goal-setting process. But it begged the question: If people who succeed have goals and those who fail have similar goals, are they essential?

Goals are commonly used in the classic New Year's resolution. I even knew a guy who kept his.

At best, goals could be seen as benign. However, they do have a few negative aspects. One of their major limitations is that they can limit performance.

Matt was training in my gym, and he wanted a program that would help him increase his bench press performance.

I developed a 12-week periodization program for the bench press in the early days of computers.

The periodization was designed to improve performance by varying the training workload or intensity over 12 weeks.

We plugged his baseline training numbers into my primitive computer program and devised a plan. He told me he was stuck or plateaued at 345 pounds; his goal was 365.

And again, a classic problem with goals: they set limits.

I suggested to Matt that we don't even pick a goal; we just choose the appropriate routine. The computer will generate the necessary workload and process, and we'll see where it leads us.

I also knew one other thing, and it's very common: Matt was overtraining.

The periodization schedule would slow him down for a few weeks and then increase his workload at the right time.

At the end of the 12-week program, he topped out at 380, much better than his targeted 365. He forgot about goals and locked into the process, a system.

And by the way, he was frustrated throughout the process because, as he told me, "I didn't feel like I was doing anything; this was way too easy."

In my 45+ years of consistent fitness, I've used a system. A commitment, along with a habit strategy, to do one simple thing: to be intentionally active every day.

Systems built on habits produce slow, steady, incremental improvements. Keep doing, keep chopping, and let the chips fall where they may.

James Clear states, "You don't rise to the level of your goals; you fall to the level of your systems."

In an interview, my son Jerry, an All-American pole vaulter at USC, was asked if he was intimidated when the bar was 18 feet high? He said no, "It only feels 8 feet high, because that's where it was set when I first started jumping, and I've kept moving it up bit by bit. I have the same feeling I had when I jumped 8 feet."

How do you get to Carnegie Hall? Process, process, process.

5.

FIND THE PERFECT COACH.

> "Half this game is 90% mental."
>
> —Phillies Manager Danny Ozark

A good coach is a supporter and cares about you beyond the game and the season.

I was extremely lucky in the coaching department. My high school football coach, Jerry Bell, guided and directed me. He made me accountable and taught me how to problem-solve.

Before high school, I bounced around between relatives and 16 different schools, and I desperately needed direction.

My college coach was cut from the same cloth. When he passed away, hundreds were there at the service, and they all had one thing in common: Each one thought they were coach John Scolinos's favorite athlete. I had to smile; I, too, thought I was his favorite.

When I went into coaching, I tried to follow the same model: stay positive, look for the good, and reinforce it. If a change needs to be made, be direct; don't make it personal.

What does that have to do with fitness consistency?

It's simply this: We all have an inner dialogue, self-talk. You are your own coach, for better or worse.

The trick is to train your inner coach, your self-talk into a positive supportive voice.

And that's exactly where I went off the rails when I started my long fitness journey. I spent time evaluating my self-talk. And remember, I was teaching this stuff, and I soon discovered that mine was negative.

What? Where in the hell did that come from? Maybe family, maybe culture? Who cares where it came from? It was there, and I needed to change it.

It was ironic because I never had coaches who used that style, and I didn't coach my athletes that way.

As I struggled and realized that this self-defeating internal dialogue was causing some of my problems, I had an epiphany.

I started pretending like I was coaching someone else. I pretended I was coaching my best friend.

Making an internal shift that is focused on encouragement and building your spirits may take time, but the rewards are enormous. Who wants to go out daily for physical activity and listen to a whining, negative voice? Nobody.

After I fired the negative coach, I started hearing some encouragement and positive feedback.

Phrases like "You can do this." "We're in this for the long haul." "The average guy wouldn't have made it to this workout, but you showed up." Or, "You did the best you could and will be back tomorrow and hit it again."

At the end of a workout, I would always give myself a verbal pat on the back. My current favorite phrase is "I'm glad I did that."

A powerful affirmation is a great reward and can go a long way in making a habit stick long-term.

6.

THE FUNDAMENTAL PRINCIPLE FOR SUCCESS IS "JUST SHOW UP."

> "A good plan violently executed now is better than a perfect plan executed next week."
>
> —General George S. Patton

Remember that university class project I talked about earlier? I, along with everyone else in the class, would present a behavior they wanted to change, explain how they went about it, and highlight one key aspect they felt made a difference.

As I evaluated my problem, I realized I struggled with consistency in my exercise program because I had created this mental image of a challenging workout that I had to do to perfection. I wasn't looking forward to it.

But I realized that once I got there, got into a light warm-up, and particularly when I controlled my intensity, things went fine. If I could only find a way to con myself into getting there and to lighten up a bit, get rid of that crazy perfectionist, "no pain, no gain" mindset.

Just get there! Just show up!

It so happened that during that semester, actor Woody Allen was quoted as saying that "90% of life was simply showing up." I heard a similar comment attributed to actress Mae West. When asked what the most important thing regarding a man in bed was, her comment was, "That he shows up."

Those quotes bounced around in my head, and something clicked. That was my solution. I needed an easy way to get to the location for the run, bike ride, workout, or hike, and once I got there, 90% of my fitness problems would be solved. Simple math, simple logic.

If I could show up, I would do something, and something would be better than nothing. If I did that consistently, I would ultimately develop a habit. That habit, over time, would lead to subtle but important changes and get me fit and healthy again.

I called it the 5-minute rule.

I made my presentation to the class. I was the professor; this better be pretty damn good.

I had developed my key concept, the 5-minute rule, based on a written commitment to show up at an exercise place five days a week for a minimum of five minutes.

My target was 30 to 45 minutes of exercise, but I could leave at the end of five minutes if I had enough. Even if I only did five minutes, I would get full credit for that workout and maintain my streak. The key was that I was in control.

It was total theory. In 1977, no one had heard of such a strategy, and when I presented the concept to many of my colleagues in the fitness world, they were skeptical. Even I was skeptical, and I'm the one who came up with it.

I gave it a shot. So far, so good.

That stupid little strategy worked, and it still works.

Over the last 45+ years, I've rarely bailed out at 5 minutes. However, the number of days I felt crappy and showed up, intending to do maybe 5 minutes, and carried on with a four-mile walk or a complete strength workout currently stands at 4,523 days. At least, that's my best guess.

When I first presented the concept in seminars and corporate workshops, the initial feedback was, "Sure, it is an excellent device to get you out to the trail or the gym. Still, I feel I would take advantage of it and become a slacker. I want to push myself and get in better shape."

However, the more feedback I received from people who successfully used the strategy, the clearer it became that the opposite was happening.

People began to tell me that once the pressure and stress of going out and doing a quad-burning hike or a long and rigorous strength training routine was lifted from their shoulders, they would find themselves pushing harder more often than not.

Another big benefit of the "just show up" strategy is that consistently showing up builds the skill of showing up! Think of showing up as building your consistency muscle.

The *Almost* in this title is the 5-minute rule. It's the glue that keeps your streak going.

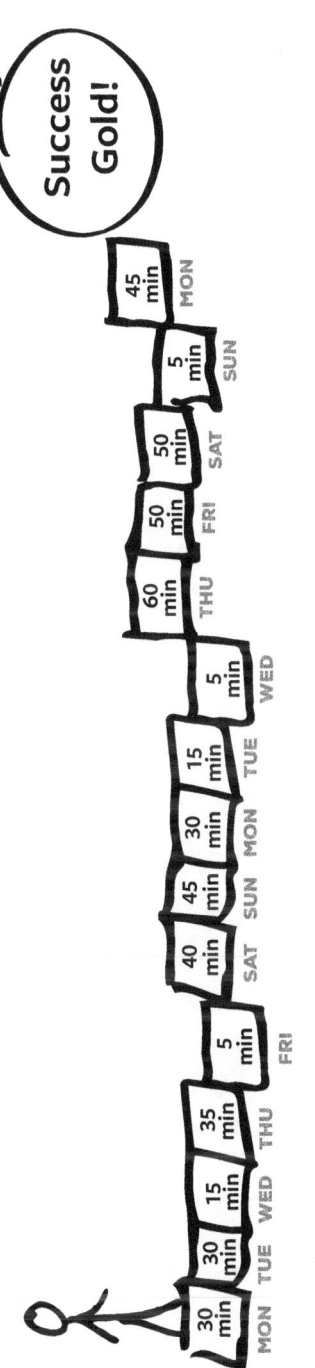

My clients would tell me that this strategy is helpful because they tended to let thoughts of a hard, gut-blasting workout or a specific distance to be run in a set time creep into their brains, resulting in procrastination.

And perfection-based thinking can suck the fun out of an otherwise enjoyable activity.

The" just show up" strategy certainly aligns with contemporary guidelines presented by James Clear, who stresses that for you to become successful in habit acquisition, you have to make it easy.

Something easy to execute, accessible, and low-friction dramatically enhances your success. It's an exercise offer that's so simple it's hard to refuse or turn down.

People have referred to the 5-minute rule as the ultimate excuse eraser: Stop whining and stressing, hold on to the habit rope, and just show up!

7.

THE WALKING BREAKTHROUGH.

It's convenient, effective, scalable, enjoyable, social, solitary, stress-reducing, can be done anywhere, and cheap. But most of all, it can become an indispensable, pleasurable habit.

> "If we were meant to walk, we'd stand upright and have two legs and opposable thumbs."
>
> —Mark Fenton

RESPECT THE WALK.

At the beginning of my fitness journey, I wasn't against walking; I just didn't consider it an actual fitness activity.

The exercise bike was the cardiovascular activity I often suggested to my clients.

I trained Scott for a couple of years. He used an exercise bike for his cardio work, and we strength trained three days a week.

His training objective was typical. He was a former D1 football player who simply wanted to get back into better shape and be consistent with his exercise routine.

His business was growing, and he traveled extensively. However, the most remarkable aspect of his life was that he was stressed to the max.

He would try to find a hotel with a fitness center, but that was not always possible.

The most problematic aspect of his business trips was the stress: the never-ending lunch meetings, dinner meetings, deadlines, and tight schedules, followed by more stress.

It became clear that the difficulty of finding a convenient training place and all the other things he had to deal with in his schedule always threw him off track.

Let's just say it was rare for Scott to maintain any semblance of a fitness routine when he took his business trips.

And that wasn't the worst of it. Typically, when Scott missed four or five days on a trip, he was pretty beat up when he returned.

I would get the call, "I'm going to need to cancel Friday's session." That cancellation would lead to a few more cancellations, and before you knew it, we might have a four- or five-week gap.

Scott made it clear that he wanted to continue to pay for his spot in my schedule because he was confident that he would be able to get back into the rhythm of things soon.

Ultimately, I would get the call, and we'd get going again. We had a pattern, and we spent a lot of time talking about how to improve his routine's on-off aspect.

The first issue was obvious: the unfamiliar travel territory, combined with all the stuff going on during his trip, threw him off. When he returned, he started dogging himself for not eating well and feeling guilty about missing his exercise.

He ultimately got back on the horse, but he felt like the horse was losing ground.

One day he was working out and mentioned that he and his wife were going on a day hike in a couple of weeks.

I could tell he wasn't looking forward to the hike, not so much because he didn't want to hike, but because he was aware that he might not have the conditioning.

He admitted that he enjoyed doing the strength training, but the cardio bike thing he had been doing before the workout was hit-or-miss and not his thing.

That and the reality that his wife was a cardiovascular fanatic.

I suggested that instead of riding his bike, or in his case, his fantasy bike routine, he take a brisk walk around the neighborhood for half an hour or so before I stop by for the next workout session.

He lived in a beautiful area with lots of rolling hills, and I tried to convince him that walking briskly in the hills would give him a good cardio workout.

I then had an idea of how to push this process along. A nearby regional park, maybe 5 minutes away, had a small trail system and was a pleasant place to walk.

"I'll meet you at that park for our next workout and walk with you. We'll pick a good pace, and I'm confident you'll get some training effect. When we're done, we'll buzz back to your house and do a condensed strength training session, maybe 30 minutes, and we'll be good.

"I just want you to get a feel for a more consistent cardio experience. If you have the hike coming up, it might be a way to train for it." The specificity of training is real.

As we were walking, I could throw in the talk test unobtrusively.

That test is a simple way to measure or evaluate the intensity level of your physical activity. It can effectively determine if you're in Zone 2 training. In Zone 2, your heart rate is between 60 and 70% of its age-based maximum rate.

You should still be able to converse when you're in that elevated heart rate Zone. If you're going up a hill, you might feel slightly out of breath, but you can still keep your sentences flowing. Most importantly, you're getting a training effect.

So off we went, with Scott clearly in Zone 2.

The talk test. Check.

When we got back to the house, I asked him how that brief hike felt, and the best I could get out of him was, "It wasn't bad."

Even though his comment was somewhat reserved, I could hear just a slight tickle of enjoyment in his voice. "Let's do this walk with a condensed strength training session for the rest of the week."

By now, you can see where this thing is headed. The weekend with his wife went well, and he continued to want to walk with the condensed strength training format.

I liked it because I was getting some activity on his dime, and something weird was happening slowly. I slowly began adding a walk into my routine when I wasn't training Scott.

But this story is so memorable because we still had the conundrum of Scott and his business trips.

When the next one came up, I suggested, "Why don't you just stick to this walking thing on these trips, whether it's a treadmill at the hotel or outside?"

He said he'd give it a shot, and it worked. When he returned, he got right back on track.

A significant breakthrough for Scott came when he realized that his walks greatly mitigated the stress of his meetings. It was an incredible stress buster.

Typically, he would have a presentation to give, and he found that ideas started to pop up on the walk. He would take a piece of paper and jot down a few critical thoughts, and overall, he's gone from hater to lover of the simple walk.

That, and the fact that he felt like he had maintained the continuity of his exercise program, made it easy for him to flow right back into his regular workout routine when he got home.

This almost accidental process that I wandered into with Scott caused me to begin thinking of walking as the perfect, simple, consistent fitness program foundation.

Like so many things in teaching, you learn from your students. I improved as a fitness coach and learned to respect the walk.

THE TOP 8 REASONS WHY WALKING WORKS FOR MOST PEOPLE MOST OF THE TIME.

1. IT'S LEGIT FITNESS.

The American College of Sports Medicine States, "Research shows that moderate physical activity, such as 30 minutes a day of brisk walking, significantly contributes to longevity."

I realize this book targets folks who've been in shape before. By this point, you've been fit and understand the benefits of cardiovascular training.

You're aware that the talk test I gave to Scott as we briskly walked through the regional park showed that he was functioning quite well and in Zone 2 of his cardiovascular training.

Longevity specialist Dr. Peter Attia stresses the importance of Zone 2 training and says most of your cardiovascular training should be in Zone 2.

Dr Attia points out that relatively moderate Zone 2 training is highly beneficial. It's easy to do, and the advantages are enormous.

No question that increasing the workload to incorporate higher levels of training can be beneficial in athletic training. However, relentless moderation in Zone 2 is the cornerstone of a basic fitness program.

2. IT'S THERAPEUTIC FOR THE BODY.

"Walk it off" is a common phrase in sports. When you're not truly injured but picked up a ding on the playing field and need to recover, you "walk it off," make an assessment, and most of the time, you're good to go.

And when you just got out of surgery, although it's been an ordeal, the physician most likely wants to get you walking as soon as possible.

That's a relatively new concept in medical treatment. Years ago, people were kept in bed for long periods until medical researchers realized that getting someone up and walking as soon as appropriate was the key to a healthy recovery.

Competitive runners often use walking as an optional training modality because it's easier on the joints.

In many ways, walking and a strength training program is the Fountain of Youth.

How you walk, your posture, and the so-called spring in your step is, to a great degree, your functional age.

If someone is surprised by your age, and I mean in a good way, I'm betting that it largely depends on how you carry yourself when you walk.

So, walk tall. It should feel like a string is attached to the top of your head, pulling you slightly upward.

Do not aggressively lean forward or back, but use a comfortable chin-up body position, looking ahead, not down at your feet.

When you have the right forward gaze, you can still see your feet but also see out in front. Pull your shoulders back a touch and have a natural arm swing.

So there, I've taken a good 15 years off your appearance.

You get my point: Walking regularly and with good posture does a body good.

3. IT'S CHEAP.

There are no membership fees or fancy equipment. Just go out the door and start walking.

That being said, don't go cheap on your shoes. Find a specialty running shoe store and get a good fitting. These stores cater to the running crowd, but more and more customers come from folks who walk as part of their fitness routine.

Remember to have a water bottle on board or back at your vehicle when you're done. The best beverage during a walk is also cheap: water. You're welcome.

And one last item: Don't go cheap on medical advice for foot care. Get the appropriate help at the first sign of an issue to keep you in the game.

The mantra I give for this is, "Keep your wheels healthy."

4. IT HAS A HIGH DO-ABILITY INDEX.

In the fitness domain, there's nothing more doable than snagging an opportunity to sneak a walk into your day.

The time it takes to get there, do it, and get back is your total transaction time for the activity.

For instance, a one-hour gym session may take over an hour and a half to complete. There's the drive to the facility, the check-in, the wardrobe change. It all adds up.

Nothing beats walking in terms of transaction time and scheduling simplicity.

5. IT'S LIKE MENTAL, DUDE.

I was turned on to the mental health and stress reduction benefits of walking long before I started walking as part of my fitness routine.

One of my friends, a counseling psychologist at the Student Health Center at the university where I was teaching, mentioned to me that, in his opinion, over 50% of the students he interacted with could greatly improve their mental health if they would just take a 30–to 45-minute walk every day.

If someone's suffering from clinical depression, they should seek professional help, but if it's stress you're dealing with, walking can be magic.

I read a heartbreaking story about a physician who lost his 12-year-old son in a tragic accident. His son was innocently playing in the field and came in contact with some discarded military explosives.

As his father told the story of this unthinkable experience, he mentioned that without his love of running, he wasn't sure if he would have made it. His ability to run helped him work through the toughest times.

Most of us have taken a walk to cool off from an emotional situation, or we're stuck on a problem we're trying to think through. We take a walk, and the solution magically pops into our heads.

When you consistently walk, you experience a relaxed, pleasant, and creative mind space. It's movement and meditation all in one.

Pacing or walking during an important phone call is second nature to most of us. Something about the movement, the relaxed stroll, makes the conversation flow.

Public speakers, rappers, and old-school preachers stroll upon the stage as they speak, as if it gives a rhythm to their thought process and boosts their memory.

As you start a regular walking program, this mental/creative benefit may play a small role, but slowly, you build your ability to let your mind wander. Ultimately, it's the biggest hook that keeps most of us going in our walking habit.

Somebody told me, "I'd like to walk, but I'm not in great spirits. When I get it together, I'll do that walking thing."

Of course, I had to tell them that's just the opposite of how it goes. You walk into a better frame of mind, a better spirit.

6. IT'S SCALABLE.

Getting up early in the morning to climb one of Colorado's 14ers, Longs Peak, or taking a stroll in the afternoon along the beach have one thing in common: walking.

A common misconception is that walking is not rigorous enough for a fitness workout. Nothing could be further from the truth. It's scalable.

Want to make walking more challenging? Try rucking.

Rucking is an activity where you carry a light load in a pack to increase the intensity.

Several NFL and NBA players use rucking in their preseason training.

Military training also relies on rucking.

The load in your rucksack doesn't need to be heavy to have a training effect; a common mistake is carrying too much weight. Doing so can change your posture and create orthopedic issues.

Another way to increase the rigor of your walk is to pick up the pace and walk more briskly. A coaching tip I often give is to walk like you're late for an appointment. Another popular line is, "Walk like you stole it."

You have to be vigilant and stay aware of your walking pace. If you're like me, your pace can unconsciously drop off throughout your walk. If you have this problem, a fun way to fix it is to play some tunes with about 140+ beats per minute. Several popular playlists feature music designed for a good walking pace.

Another great way to increase intensity is to find a walk with various steep grades. There should be many slow, gradual grades with a few short, steep sections mixed in. I call that a HIIT (High Intensity Interval Training) trail.

My favorite method of increasing intensity is to find a long set of stairs or steps along my walking path. Depending on how long they are, I may do a series of repeats and then resume my walk.

The most common form of this activity is seen in stadiums, where groups of athletes walk or run stadium stairs.

Brendan Leonard's book, *I Hate Running, and You Can Too*, has a chapter entitled, "Walking is Running." He explains that for most people running a marathon, walking is critical to their strategy. One thing that's never asked of someone who completes a marathon is, "Did you walk at all?" It's not relevant.

At some point in his walking and running career, Brendan began running ultramarathons—serious stuff: 50 mile races, 100 mile races. He said that when people mention they could never run that far, he replies, "I can't either. Almost nobody does. We walk. Some of us walk a lot."

By the way, it's perfectly legal for a walker to break into an occasional jog. Many walkers use this strategy.

In that sense, runners and walkers are in the same family. It's just that I see more walkers smiling than I ever see runners smile. Undoubtedly, runners are smiling on the inside.

7. IT'S VERSATILE, STEALTHY, AND HEALTHY.

Is walking with a friend, a small group, or solo better? One of the things I love about walking is its versatility.

Walking with a friend or a small group can be a great experience, but my most common approach is to go solo. The reasons are simple: There is no planning, and I can keep my pace to maintain my fitness.

Another benefit of going solo is that if you think scheduling can be challenging, imagine how hard it is to get two schedules or more to mesh.

We have a new phenomenon: More and more people are doing their work remotely rather than in person.

The Health Enhancement Research Organization (HERO) reports on a Stanford study showing that remote workers sit two more hours per day than in-person workers. Walking is a perfect solution. Take five 10- to 15-minute walk breaks a day. Use a reminder app and make it happen.

8. IT'S ENJOYABLE.

The undeniable growth of walking for fitness and pleasure is based on one fundamental fact: It can be enjoyable, something you look forward to.

From the brisk morning walk that wakes up the systems and makes for a better day to a casual stroll with a friend, walking has always been a part of daily life for humans.

For the last 70 years, the automobile has taken over and made walking seem like a negative experience. The general feeling has been that successful people ride, while walking is for the elderly and those without a car.

Thankfully, some people have rediscovered the most organic of fitness activities.

People have discovered the joy and benefits of walking and have built their wardrobes around their walking activity. Comfortable athletic shoes and breathable fabrics help people to be ready to go at a moment's notice.

Some health-conscious athletes are ditching the golf cart and walking the course. There is a growing trend of prestigious destination golf courses that are walking only.

When someone asks my friend Dan Alfieri why he chose to walk the course, his answer is simple: "Because I can!"

Walking, particularly carrying your own clubs, is a legitimate fitness activity. Walking over 18 holes can be a six- or seven-mile trek.

Contrary to the saying "golf is a good walk spoiled," it isn't. Particularly if you're doing it with good friends and don't three-putt.

Vacations can also be built around walking. Walking tours are available in Ireland or Switzerland, and tourist attractions all over the United States offer them too.

Comedian Adam Carolla says he gets out and hoofs it whenever he gets to a new town. He explains that that's the only way you get to know the place.

When it's all said and done, the real reason walking has exploded is simple. People feel better, and they enjoy it.

BOB MULLIGAN'S EIGHT SIMPLE STEPS TO ALMOST CONSISTENT FITNESS.

1. Just Show Up. A healthy smoothie is waiting for you when you're done.

2. Do a fitness activity for at least 5 minutes, hopefully longer.

3. Pretend you're going to enjoy it.

4. Find your pace and keep going. You can stop or change the intensity at any time.

5. Keep going. You're starting to feel okay—pretty good, actually. You've got this.

6. Wind down and bring it on in. You feel energized and relaxed. It's fun to succeed.

7. Enjoy the smoothie.

8. Repeat Tomorrow . . . Probably.

8.

WALKING STRATEGIES—A PRACTICAL GUIDE.

SHOULD I WALK FOR A CERTAIN AMOUNT OF TIME OR A CERTAIN DISTANCE?

I suggest using time as your target rather than distance.

First of all, distance can vary significantly depending on the terrain. A rugged three-mile hike at elevation could be pretty tough, whereas a 3-mile hike on flat terrain would be quite easy.

I've always gone out for a certain amount of time rather than a particular distance. First and foremost, I'm like everybody else; I have a schedule to keep.

Another benefit of walking for time rather than distance is that it makes it a low-pressure activity.

Some days, I may feel full of energy and want to pick up the pace, but then, I can take it down a notch to a comfortable stroll on another day.

However, if you decide to walk, let's say 5 miles, yet you're pressed for time, the only way you could make it is if you bust your butt. That's a lot of pressure and something you might not look forward to.

SHOULD I USE A STEP COUNTER?

Measuring steps has been around for a while.

According to Wikipedia, in 1777, Abraham-Louis Perrelet built a device that could measure your walking distance. A few years later, in 1960, a Japanese professor sold a device that measured steps, and he set an ideal target of approximately 5 miles, 10,000 steps.

The 10,000-step idea has been criticized because it is not based on science. The whole deal is considered fairly arbitrary and a marketing gimmick.

I accept that that's true, but over the last number of years, in real-life experience, I found for myself and my clients that 10,000–15,000 steps per day is a good target for most people, most of the time.

I do have one reservation about step counting, which I'll talk about later.

I don't know many folks without some form of step counter. For many of us, there's a counter built into our phones, although that has some limitations on daily step counting because you don't always have your phone with you.

You might have a Fitbit or an Apple Watch. You can also buy a cheap step counter on Amazon that works just fine.

The step counter has been a big breakthrough in encouraging people to add activity to their lives. It provides some objectivity to help answer the question, "How active am I during my day?"

You may have walked 11,000 steps during the day and found that your sleep quality was much better than usual.

It can give you a baseline, an awareness of how much you move during your day, and help you move from sedentary to unsedentary.

As you begin your fitness walking program, I would like you to put walking into two buckets.

You have a scheduled daily intentional fitness walk in one bucket, which might take 15 minutes to an hour. This planned, intentional fitness session gives you both physiological and mental benefits. It's a consistent daily fitness activity you can count on. It's where the magic happens.

In the other bucket, you accrue steps throughout your day. These steps are a function of looking for opportunities to get more movement into your life.

Medicine & Science in Sports & Exercise research shows that any physical activity, regardless of duration, has benefits, including reducing all-cause mortality.

In other words, those incidental steps during the day count.

I affectionately call those incidental steps my side hustle or my junk steps.

Being aware of this incidental activity, those junk steps, if you will, throughout my day encourages me to look for creative ways to add movement.

For instance, I commonly carry groceries in from the car and realize I don't need to load up. I can make as many trips back and forth as I want because it adds more movement to my day.

You should park at the far end of a parking lot for two reasons: there will be no door dings, and you won't have to circle to find the closest spot because you're an athlete.

Avoid elevators and hunt for the staircase whenever you have a few floors to climb.

But remember that although step counting is a great tool, relying on the total number of steps doesn't always give you an accurate picture. It can only give you a general snapshot.

The steps you take on a steep mountain trail or steps up stadium stairs are more rigorous than those of walking or strolling from one store to the next on a shopping trip.

A day you do 9,000 steps may feel more challenging than a day you do 15,000.

The American College of Sports Medicine published a chart developed by C Tudor-Locke and DR Bassett (2004) that categorizes the number of daily steps in relation to activity levels.

Number of Steps	Activity Level
0–5,000	Sedentary
5,000–7,499	Low Active
7,500–9,999	Somewhat Active
10,000–12,500	Active
12,500 or more	Highly Active

Okay, here's that reservation I talked about earlier. Steps are fantastic for gaining awareness of your overall activity level. It's quantifiable, but that quantification can also become the enemy.

I heard somebody say that if you want to kill the fun in anything, you should start quantifying it or putting numbers on it.

I encourage people to check their step count once or twice weekly to look back and see their trends. The step number I like people to focus on is their monthly average.

The critical issue in quantifying numbers is monitoring yourself. If you feel step counting is adding stress to your life, you might consider putting it on the back burner for a while.

But if you modify your obsession, reflect on your patterns, stay curious, and examine how you feel, step counting can be a real benefit.

On a personal note, I have a magic number of steps that make me feel right at the end of the day. I know I've hit the mark if I fall asleep quickly and comfortably.

EXCUSE ME, DID YOU JUST FARTLEK?

If you didn't, it's certainly something I would recommend.

When I was a track coach, nothing got the giggles going more than when I introduced the concept of fartlek training to new runners coming out for the track team. The veteran runners didn't giggle; they simply looked forward to an enjoyable running workout.

The term fartlek is a Swedish word that means speed play. It's been used over the years to train runners with the primary intent of keeping things interesting.

Rather than a standard interval training session, where you run a specific distance in a specific time, with a specific interval of rest, the fartlek training method allows the athletes to take off on a run and improvise as they go.

The athletes are on their own to alternate easy jogging with periods of sprinting and cruising, improvising all based on how they feel in the moment.

The athletes loved it because it was playful and virtually eliminated the boring workout.

I use the fartlek walk technique nearly daily on my fitness walks. Stop giggling.

I might start with an easy stroll, then pick my pace up and have a good rhythm. At some point, I pick a target—often a telephone pole off in the distance or some other visual—and put it into high gear to see how quickly I can reach that point.

Then I gear down into a comfortable pace again and continue to play with my speed the whole time.

The fundamental premise of this type of training is that you don't have a grueling workout hanging over your head; you're in control.

So get out there and fartlek to your heart's desire.

AT WHAT ELEVATION DOES WALKING TURN INTO HIKING?

Did you take a walk or go on a hike?

It's an ongoing debate. How do you differentiate between walking and hiking?

According to experts, the most common difference is that hiking is on a dirt path or trail, and walking is on pavement.

The image of the hiker is one of backpacks, granola, and an earthy fragrance. The typical daily fitness hiker may have none of these.

My theory is that walking is hiking when you say it is. It just sounds more athletic and challenging. Maybe it's a guy thing—I'm always looking for street cred, or in this case, trail cred.

I enjoy walking a dirt trail. It's out in nature, and the uneven surface of the trail helps me maintain my balance and strength. My brief daily fitness hike involves walking; I mean hiking. Okay, now I'm even confused.

It's simply good, consistent exercise—forget about the name.,

EARBUDS OR A NAKED WALK?

> "My walk is my game. It's a therapeutic dance. It's a creativity lab. I even have my own walk-up music."
>
> —RPM

The complaint that exercise is boring was virtually eliminated in 1979 by the advent of the Walkman, followed by iPods in 2001 and the AirPod in 2016.

Technology has improved dramatically, and you can enjoy a podcast while maintaining awareness of the sounds around you. When

I ask people what gets them out and exercising, many tell me they've bundled their favorite podcast with their daily activities.

The key is a bundling hook. You don't listen to your favorite podcast unless you're out for a walk or in the gym working out.

You can enjoy the pleasure of listening to your favorite music or laughing while listening to your favorite comedian.

But I also cherish a nature vibe without AirPods being plugged into my head.

I refer to this as walking naked. I've heard others refer to it as silent walking. Whatever the name, there are incredible advantages.

It lets me sort things out, prioritize projects, generate creative thoughts, and enjoy quiet and pleasant internal conversations.

When people ask me how to make exercise enjoyable, my first answer is to get some AirPods, listen to a podcast you enjoy, and be on your way.

But never underestimate the pleasure you can get if you find the right location and walk naked.

THE TREADMILL.

By this point in the book, you realize I'm a guy who loves walking in natural landscapes. It can be a path in the park, a mountain trail, along the river, or on a beach.

But I'm also a guy who has committed to exercising every day, and like all of us, I have days when things don't come together.

It might be the weather, a series of back-to-back meetings, or a rescheduled appointment that's destroyed your daily schedule. Whatever the circumstances, you've reached the latter part of your day, and your exercise streak is in serious jeopardy.

Days like these are streak-busters.

Consistent exercisers know these days happen and have contingency plans.

The best solution for most people is to have a home cardio piece available.

You may already have an exercise piece and have used it for other purposes. Well, dust it off and put that thing into action. It might be an exercise bike, an elliptical, a rower, or a treadmill. It's what I call the ultimate excuse eraser.

My favorite is a basic but well-made treadmill.

It doesn't need a lot of programming features or bells and whistles; you just want a solid, dependable machine.

While some exercise machines have come and gone over the years, the treadmill will always be used to maintain fitness.

And there's something that makes the treadmill unique, different from other cardiovascular devices like the bike, the rowing machine, or the elliptical. The treadmill gently pulls you along at whatever speed you set. It may be set at a slow speed, but you will walk.

The walk isn't a happy walk for a minute or two, but then you get a rhythm, and you're watching a TV show or listening to a podcast while exercising, and your mood picks up.

Unlike a bike, a rower, or an elliptical, where each stroke requires a thoughtful effort, walking on a treadmill can become comfortably mindless. I mean, you need to be aware of your surroundings from a safety standpoint, but there's something relaxing about the rhythm of walking on the treadmill.

Here are two steps you should consider taking before purchasing a treadmill.

The first step might be to join a fitness club, particularly one with a trial membership. That would allow you to use a treadmill to see if it is something you can commit to and use.

There is nothing unethical about that strategy. You may decide to join.

But for those familiar with the treadmill who already acknowledge it would be a great addition to their fitness arsenal, the next step to consider is finding a local specialty fitness store.

Specialty fitness stores have a variety of brands on the floor and allow you to try them out. The other biggie is that specialty fitness stores have a service component to their business. In other words, if you have a problem, they can fix it.

Another popular option, and one that can save you a few bucks, is to search Facebook Marketplace for a used high-quality treadmill.

I'm trying to keep my advice low-key, and it *is* possible to maintain a walking habit without access to a treadmill. But I would be less than honest if I didn't let you know that my habit of walking, my substantial streak, would have been much harder without my treadmill. It's always there for me.

CREATE A LOW-FRICTION WALK ENVIRONMENT. KNOW THE TERRITORY.

You know the rule by now: the lower the friction you encounter while trying to maintain a habit, the higher the likelihood of success.

We also know from research presented by Katy Milkman in her excellent book, *How to Change*, that people with flexible schedules succeed more in their fitness routines. They stay aware of when and where a fitness opportunity may appear in their schedule.

They also know the territory.

There may be a park on your way to an appointment, and you leave 20 to 30 minutes early because the freeway traffic is unknowable, and you don't want to be late.

But there was no traffic, and you arrived 20 to 30 minutes early. There's a walking trail nearby, and you can grab a quick 15 minutes.

Develop a fitness opportunity map in your mind. Think of your walking program as an activity that constantly seeks opportunities.

How many days a week should I train?

The conventional wisdom was to start people slowly with, say, three days per week and then gradually increasing the workout time—ultimately, adding a day or two more into the schedule.

I've tried that with many folks and realized it was extremely difficult for people to add more days to their schedules. Once they locked into 3 days a week, they stayed at 3 days a week.

The interesting thing was that when I experimented with having people work out five days a week right from the start, and kept their time per workout to a very modest number, say 20 minutes, five days a week—their consistency was better than that of the people who started with a three-day-per-week/30-minute-per-session approach.

It became clear that it's a lot easier to add time to a five-day-a-week schedule than to add days to a three-day-a-week schedule.

The other thing to consider in our 5-day-a-week plan is that we're developing a foundation with fitness walking. Fitness walking doesn't require a lot of transaction time. It's doable at a moment's notice.

THE OPTION THAT'S EASIER THAN YOU THINK—NO DAYS OFF.

Bill Belichick and the Patriots used this slogan, but I've used it in my routine for many years.

Initially, I had a pretty standard five-day workout routine.

I would do my strength training and cardio on Monday, Tuesday, Thursday, and Friday. On Wednesday, I would focus on cardio training. My rest days were pretty classic: Saturday and Sunday.

But I realized that I looked forward to Saturday and Sunday for no reason. I was feeling great about my five-day-a-week program, but it was almost as if I had created some negativity about the days I worked out.

It was clear that there was a simple solution: make Saturday and Sunday low-key movement days, something light and easy. Make exercise an everyday activity, a way of life, something you do daily, sort of like breathing.

Another way to think of it is that by adopting a seven-day-a-week plan, you've created a situation where you have one less decision to make every day. You remove the decision of whether or not to work out.

Performing an action unconsciously is what psychologists call automaticity, an effortless execution of a task through repetition or practice.

Doing an activity every day can enhance automaticity. Writers and musicians have known this for years. They realize that no matter what, they will spend some time everyday writing, composing, or practicing.

It may not be a lengthy session, but they know when they get up in the morning that at some point during their day, they're going to work at their craft. It might only be 15 minutes, but they know it strengthens their skills.

The first topic often discussed in this conversation is overtraining and the need for rest days. To some degree, that's true, particularly for high-performance athletes pushing their limits.

But I've known several high-performance athletes who work out seven days a week and solve the problem of overtraining by having days they call active rest. An active rest day may be nothing more than some stretching and a walk.

For most people who take a relatively light approach to fitness training, 45 minutes of walking seven days a week and 30 minutes of strength training three days a week should be enough to handle that without any concerns about overtraining.

If you experience classic signs of overtraining, such as trouble falling asleep, feeling out of gas, and having no energy, simply reduce the amount of time or intensity in your routine.

My suggestion would also be to check with your doctor and see if you may have a health issue you're struggling with.

Simplify your life; no days off.

I'M SO GLAD I DID THIS—THE REWARD.

> "It doesn't matter how slowly you go as long as you do not stop."
>
> —Confucius

Rewards are more effective when they're linked to the activity. In other words, they are not sent off in the distant future but rather tied to the moment after your exercise session.

I always ask my clients how they feel as we conclude a session and they're in their cool-down period.

They tell me how good they feel as their bodies relax after a session, and the endorphin release is evident. They also mention a burst of energy for a substantial period of time after they've exercised.

An area of reward is also the whole idea of self-efficacy—the satisfaction you get when you've accomplished something previously difficult. You kept your commitment; you're succeeding.

Beyond the good feeling you have after your workout or the self-efficacy, a treat never hurts.

Maybe something as simple as sparkling water and a slice of lime or a smoothie—I should say a healthy smoothie; there is a difference.

I also do a little mind game in the morning: When I get up, I won't have the desired cup of coffee until I throw the yoga mat down on the floor and do some core exercises and stretching.

Then, the coffee.

I had a client get in the best shape of his life during football season because he only watched football if he was walking on his treadmill—and he loved football.

Be creative. Always remember coffee will get you on the mat, not some distant health benefit.

9.

GETTING YOUR S**** TOGETHER... THE PLAN.

Getting your **stuff** together takes more than hope or a fired-up attitude; it takes a plan built on a strategy and a commitment. It's time to stop flirting and commit.

A COMMITMENT THAT'S SO EASY, YOU CAN'T SAY NO.

> Most people fail, not because of the lack of desire, but, because of the lack of commitment.
>
> —Vince Lombardi

You go to the gym and work out. You look in the mirror and check for any physical changes that have taken place. Zip, nada, absolutely no change.

You do the same thing every day for a few weeks, putting in the effort, but you don't see results. You haven't realized that you're feeling a little better bit by bit; you're just focused on the cosmetic stuff. And then you quit two weeks in; you had enough.

Let's pretend you have a clone, and your clone has taken a different approach. He committed to sticking with his program because he believed it would work slowly over time. Small increments of daily effort will add up to long-term success.

A commitment may seem trivial and a waste of time, silly even. I wrote a simple commitment over 45 years ago and keep it to this day. I guess I just like being silly.

In Robert Cialdini's book, *Influence*, he reviews the six principles of persuasion, and states that once we make a stand for ourselves or others we have applied pressure to behave consistently with that commitment. This is considered a soft yet powerful commitment.

A soft commitment is typically a written statement of your intentions. It can be kept private or shared with a friend.

If you choose to confide in a friend, let them know that you desire to stay committed to a consistent exercise plan and appreciate their support.

Also, let them know that you've struggled with what you're taking on and have no expectations of perfection.

A hard commitment is like wearing a goofy costume if you fail to keep it or carrying a sign through the office announcing that you've quit your exercise program.

The problem with a hard commitment is that when you fail, and there's a reasonable probability that that happens, the restart is much more difficult because of all the drama associated with your previous effort.

A soft commitment slip-up is not nearly as punitive, and returning to your fitness habit after a slip-up is much easier.

Keeping your word is more potent than a joke side bet.

The strategy is straightforward: Commit to consistent activity and make it so easy that it's hard to turn down. The strength of the commitment is built on a conviction that you won't let yourself down. You may stumble at some point, but you'll get back up and recommit.

A commitment is a nudge to get active . . . even when you're not in the mood.

So whether you call it a long-term super goal, an intention, or a mission statement, a commitment is a written statement that gives you a solid platform to start your action plan.

In the next section, I will give you a sample commitment to fill out.

It's the same commitment I've used with folks over the years. It was vital in my own personal journey.

Feel free to modify or change it however you see fit. Make something that will work for you.

I also have a space for you to jot down your **why**.

You'll notice that I recommend a 5-, 6-, or 7-day-a-week schedule. I highly recommend the 7-day, no-days-off approach because it eliminates the thought process. If a day ends in Y, you exercise.

I understand that a "no days off schedule" might not appeal to you at the beginning of the process. With that in mind, you can select a five- or six-day-a-week schedule.

I'll also leave room for you to freehand your commitment here in the book.

MY FITNESS COMMITMENT.

I commit to showing up for a planned walk/fitness activity and exercise for a minimum of 5 minutes 5/6/7 days a week. My only legitimate excuse is if I'm on IR (injured reserve) or if it's a PRD (planned rest day). The days I show up and work out, or I'm on IR or a planned rest day, all count toward my streak.

Typically, my sessions last 30 to 60 minutes.

Why this commitment is vital to me:

Signed _____

Modifications:

10.

THE ALMOST CONSISTENT FITNESS STREAK TRACKER.

HOW AN AWARENESS TOOL CAN HELP YOU MAINTAIN YOUR FITNESS INVESTMENT.

Streak tracking and journaling are both excellent tools for gaining awareness and moving toward fitness success.

You can develop your own handwritten journal, use one of the many available free apps, or use our "Almost Consistent Streak Tracker." Whatever approach you decide to take, keeping a record of your activity can be very beneficial.

I might add that my favorite free app is *DAY ONE*. The *DAY ONE* app functions well as a tracker and a journaling tool. It's available for both Apple and Android devices.

So, while the DAY ONE app, or our "Streak Tracker" may be your preference, you may also find that physically writing out your record of activity improves your ability to see subtle but significant associations and, through that process, make critical course corrections.

A recent University of Tokyo study in 2021 revealed that physical writing can lead to more brain activity. Who doesn't need more brain activity?

Journaling can give you a big picture of your progress and how you're doing on many levels. It can give you trends and patterns, what's working, what's not, and why.

The bottom line: whether you use our "Almost Consistent Fitness Streak Tracker", the app , or create your own journal, you will feel accountable and aware of the investment you've made in your health and fitness.

What do I mean by investment?

An exciting way to look at the whole project is to consider your fitness consistency, your fitness streak, as an investment in you.

I would look at my fitness log and realize that I had made substantial improvements and positive changes, and like any change, it wasn't easy.

I couldn't shake the fact that if I stopped for a period of time, I knew I would lose some of that progress. I felt as if I were dumping money down the toilet.

Our simple "Almost Consistent Fitness Streak Tracker" will help you stay on course. We've designed it so that if you skip a session, we've built strategies to encourage you to get right back on track and retain the vast amount of progress you've already made.

Take pride in what you've done, and keep moving forward. You're a doer; you're still in the game. The real problem is the people who are sitting on the sidelines, watching and thinking they might want to start, but for one reason or another, they haven't. Be grateful you're not them.

A great aspect of habit tracking is that you get a clear visual of your streak, and after all, the streak is a great consistency barometer. We're aware of streaks in sports: Hitting streaks, losing streaks, three-point shot streaks, and consecutive championships. And the streaks go on and on.

The Almost Consistent Fitness approach and its 5-minute rule make it easy to keep your streak going. It's just 5 minutes. There are over 1400 minutes in a day. Gimme 5. Who doesn't have 5 minutes?

SCHEDULE SCHEDULE SCHEDULE.

For some people, scheduling their exercise session is relatively easy. Their lives are hectic and beyond busy, and they can only commit to exercise when there are no interruptions—the early morning before the chaos begins.

The energy boost you get from an early morning workout can keep you charged the whole day.

Talk about automaticity. The sun comes up, you exercise. Log your activity and move on with your day.

But for most folks, scheduling exercise is more involved. It takes flexibility and determination.

The best approach is to create a habit of scanning your schedule each morning and finding a time slot for your daily exercise.

Bring technology into the game and use a scheduling app.

When you find that golden opportunity in your schedule, don't fall into the trap of thinking you can always slide it back and do it later in the day. Do it at the first opportunity. It must have that level of priority. Learn to read on the move and when you see an opportunity do it.

Finding the time is a non-negotiable part of the daily schedule for the successful exerciser. You've committed to making exercise a part of your day, and at some point before the end of your day, you will exercise.

Popular author Scott Galloway talks about fitness as a non-negotiable investment in yourself for your enjoyment and personal enhancement. He uses a great line regarding this commitment:

"My success is my fault."

That's accountability in a nutshell.

Streaks and bounce backs.

Streaks have become an incredibly popular way to coax a long-term habit. There are an abundance of books, guides, and apps on the subject, but streaks are nothing new.

Particularly in sports, there's Joe DiMaggio's streak of getting a hit in 56 consecutive games, winning streaks, losing streaks, and every other kind of streak imaginable. When we watch a sporting event on TV, we're driven nuts by obscure streak stats generated via analytics.

The most impotant metric . . . your Almost Consistent Win Percentage.

There's a tendency for some people, when playing a streak game, to feel that if they end their streak, all is lost. The benefits and progress made during the streak are all gone. Nothing could be further from the truth. We're playing a game here, people. Sure, it should create an awareness that No-Shows have the potential of becoming another and another. But under no circumstances should you feel you've lost the game. I'd suggest you take pride in that you've made a great effort to this point in time and reset as soon as possible.

Remember, the "Almost Consistent Fitness Streak Tracker" is a game designed to help you stay as consistent as possible. There is no perfection here. That's why we call it *almost* consistent. Focus on your overall win percentage, not just your streak.

What do I mean by an overall win percentage?

Your win percentage is the number of times you showed up monthly minus the skips. From that number, you can calculate your winning percentage.

We see it all the time in sports. For instance, in Major League Baseball, a team that wins 60% of their games is considered outstanding.

In the ACF streak game, if you missed a couple of days in the month and broke your streak, those two misses would still give you an over 90% winning percentage. That, by any measure, means you're doing well. Keep the focus on the win rate and not so much on the no-shows.

THE BOUNCE BACK FACTOR.

The key to success is a quick reset after a streak has ended. If you do that in sports, you have what they call a bounce back. Teams in all sports are rated on their ability to bounce back from inevitable losses during the season. It's just the nature of sports. There's no sport called perfect.

I've used sports analogies throughout. Here's another one. Let's say the Warriors get a big lead in the first half, but in the waning minutes of the first half, they stop playing defense, start taking bad shots, and let the lead slip away. At halftime, the coach, Steve Kerr, will give his speech. "*Shake it off*, get back to *who we are*, and do the things we practice; everything else will take care of itself."

That's exactly the mindset I want you to have in the ACF streak game. *Shake it off* and *start hitting your shots*. You're better than that. End of cliches.

HOW TO USE YOUR "ALMOST CONSISTENT FITNESS STREAK TRACKER."

The "ACF Streak Tracker" guidelines:

1. Commit to a 5, 6, or 7-day schedule of intentional walking/fitness activity. Start small.

2. For the first four weeks, try to stay in the 15- to 30-minute range, then increase to 30 to 45+ as you move into the second month. But at any time, feel free to do just 5 minutes.

3. On those days when you feel compelled to do just 5 minutes, consider that those are probably the most essential workout days in your program. In the past, you might not have shown up without that option.

4. Think of the 5-minute rule as the ultimate streak saver, the game within the game.

5. If you show up, that day counts in the streak. That includes IR (injuries) and PRDs (planned rest days). You have a limit of two PRDs per week.

6. Build the longest streak possible with your daily exercise session and make it a game. If you do have a No-Show, bounce back the next.

When you see the filled-out sample of the "Streak Tracker," it will all make sense. It's straightforward and intuitive. I recommend that you use your tracker. The daily tracker and its weekly and monthly summaries can give you some real insights.

Here's an overview on how to use your "Daily Streaker Tracker."

CURRENT STREAK:
This is your third week without a miss; your streak is 21.

RECORD STREAK:
Last year, you had a streak of 97 straight, which is your best so far.

WHEN?:
Make a note of your start time when you schedule.

YOU SHOWED UP/REST DAY:
Check the box for a win when you show up, are on IR (have an injury), or took a PRD (planned rest day).

WHERE?:
This could be more than one place. It could be your walking spot and the gym.

ACTIVITY:
It could be strength training followed by a short hike.

DURATION:
Your activity is on the clock.

INTENSITY LEVELS:
   Easy—A relaxed walk with a friend, a stroll.
   Moderate/Zone 2—Hilly terrain, rucking, brisk walk, etc.
   Fartlek—A fun walk with speed changes.
   Hard—Pushing your limits.

A NO-SHOW:
Oops, so, you missed your exercise session and stopped your streak. It's no problem; do a reset and start a new streak tomorrow.

START ENERGY:
Rate your energy at the beginning of your workout: high, medium, or low.

RECOVERY ENERGY:
Rate your energy 10 minutes after you cool down at the end of your workout.

WEEKLY TOTAL EXERCISE TIME:
Target a minimum of 150 to 300 minutes of moderate to vigorous exercise per week.

WEEKLY AND MONTHLY STEP COUNT AVERAGES:
A great snapshot of your overall activity level.

MONTHLY ALMOST CONSISTENT WIN RATE %:
A simple calculation gives you a valid success rate.

NOTES:
This can be used to share any thoughts or ideas regarding your activities. You might have had a No-Show and are wondering what the trigger was or why your energy level is higher than it usually is. It's also a great place to put information about your strength training program. Or maybe track your daily steps or rate your effort to become unsedentary throughout your day. It's your space, be creative.

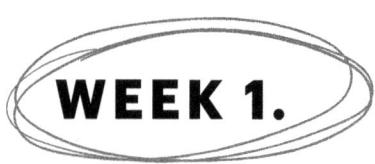
WEEK 1.

MON. 1/5 CURRENT STREAK 20

You Showed Up/Rest Day ☒ **INTENSITY**
When? _7 a.m._ ☐ Easy
Where? _Redrock Trail_ ☐ Moderate/Zone2
Activity _Walk_ ☒ Fartlek
☐ Hard

Start Energy ↑ →⊗(↓)   Recovery Energy (↑)→ ↓
Duration _40 min_   You No-Showed ☐
(Oops, Reset Tomorrow)

NOTES:
Felt strong—bump it up to 45 on Wednesday.

TUE. 1/6 CURRENT STREAK 21

You Showed Up/Rest Day ☒ **INTENSITY**
When? _6 p.m._ ☐ Easy
Where? _Gym_ ☒ Moderate/Zone2
Activity _Tread/Weights_ ☐ Fartlek
☐ Hard

Start Energy ↑(→)↓   Recovery Energy (↑)→ ↓
Duration _1 hr_   You No-Showed ☐
(Oops, Reset Tomorrow)

NOTES:
15 min on treadmill @ 3.9-2% grade good.
Squat form needs work.

12-WEEK ~~ALMOST~~ CONSISTENT STREAK TRACKER

WEEK 1.

MON. / CURRENT STREAK ___

You Showed Up/Rest Day ☐   **INTENSITY**
When? _____   ☐ Easy
Where? _____   ☐ Moderate/Zone2
Activity _____   ☐ Fartlek
                                                 ☐ Hard

Start Energy ↑ → ↓   Recovery Energy ↑ → ↓

Duration _____   You No-Showed ☐
                                                 (Oops, Reset   Tomorrow)

NOTES:

TUE. / CURRENT STREAK ___

You Showed Up/Rest Day ☐   **INTENSITY**
When? _____   ☐ Easy
Where? _____   ☐ Moderate/Zone2
Activity _____   ☐ Fartlek
                                                 ☐ Hard

Start Energy ↑ → ↓   Recovery Energy ↑ → ↓

Duration _____   You No-Showed ☐
                                                 (Oops, Reset   Tomorrow)

NOTES:

WED. / CURRENT STREAK ___

You Showed Up/Rest Day ☐   **INTENSITY**
When? _____   ☐ Easy
Where? _____   ☐ Moderate/Zone2
Activity _____   ☐ Fartlek
   ☐ Hard

Start Energy ↑ → ↓   Recovery Energy ↑ → ↓

Duration _____   You No-Showed ☐
   (Oops, Reset Tomorrow)

NOTES:

THU. / CURRENT STREAK ___

You Showed Up/Rest Day ☐   **INTENSITY**
When? _____   ☐ Easy
Where? _____   ☐ Moderate/Zone2
Activity _____   ☐ Fartlek
   ☐ Hard

Start Energy ↑ → ↓   Recovery Energy ↑ → ↓

Duration _____   You No-Showed ☐
   (Oops, Reset Tomorrow)

NOTES:

FRI. / CURRENT STREAK ___

You Showed Up/Rest Day ☐   **INTENSITY**
When? _____   ☐ Easy
Where? _____   ☐ Moderate/Zone2
Activity _____   ☐ Fartlek
                                    ☐ Hard

Start Energy ↑ → ↓   Recovery Energy ↑ → ↓

Duration _____   You No-Showed ☐
                                    (Oops, Reset Tomorrow)

NOTES:

SAT. / CURRENT STREAK ___

You Showed Up/Rest Day ☐   **INTENSITY**
When? _____   ☐ Easy
Where? _____   ☐ Moderate/Zone2
Activity _____   ☐ Fartlek
                                    ☐ Hard

Start Energy ↑ → ↓   Recovery Energy ↑ → ↓

Duration _____   You No-Showed ☐
                                    (Oops, Reset Tomorrow)

NOTES:

SUN. / CURRENT STREAK ___

You Showed Up/Rest Day ☐
When? _____
Where? _____
Activity _____

INTENSITY
☐ Easy
☐ Moderate/Zone2
☐ Fartlek
☐ Hard

Start Energy ↑ → ↓

Duration _____

Recovery Energy ↑ → ↓

You No-Showed ☐
(Oops, Reset Tomorrow)

NOTES:

WEEKLY SUMMARY

CURRENT STREAK ___
RECORD STREAK ___

Total Days You Showed Up/Rest Days _____
Total Days You No-Showed _____
Total Exercise Time _____
Weekly Step Avg. _____

NOTES:

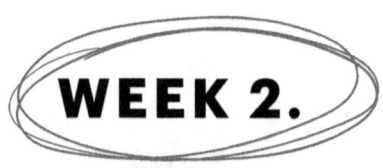

WEEK 2.

MON. / CURRENT STREAK ___

You Showed Up/Rest Day ☐   **INTENSITY**
When? _____ ☐ Easy
Where? _____ ☐ Moderate/Zone2
Activity _____ ☐ Fartlek
                                            ☐ Hard

Start Energy ↑ → ↓   Recovery Energy ↑ → ↓

Duration _____   You No-Showed ☐
                                      (Oops, Reset Tomorrow)

NOTES:

TUE. / CURRENT STREAK ___

You Showed Up/Rest Day ☐   **INTENSITY**
When? _____ ☐ Easy
Where? _____ ☐ Moderate/Zone2
Activity _____ ☐ Fartlek
                                            ☐ Hard

Start Energy ↑ → ↓   Recovery Energy ↑ → ↓

Duration _____   You No-Showed ☐
                                      (Oops, Reset Tomorrow)

NOTES:

WED. / CURRENT STREAK ___

You Showed Up/Rest Day ☐ **INTENSITY**
When? _____ ☐ Easy
Where? _____ ☐ Moderate/Zone2
Activity _____ ☐ Fartlek
☐ Hard

Start Energy ↑ → ↓   Recovery Energy ↑ → ↓

Duration _____ You No-Showed ☐
(Oops, Reset   Tomorrow)

NOTES:

THU. / CURRENT STREAK ___

You Showed Up/Rest Day ☐ **INTENSITY**
When? _____ ☐ Easy
Where? _____ ☐ Moderate/Zone2
Activity _____ ☐ Fartlek
☐ Hard

Start Energy ↑ → ↓   Recovery Energy ↑ → ↓

Duration _____ You No-Showed ☐
(Oops, Reset   Tomorrow)

NOTES:

FRI. /   CURRENT STREAK ___

You Showed Up/Rest Day ☐   **INTENSITY**
When? _____   ☐ Easy
Where? _____   ☐ Moderate/Zone2
Activity _____   ☐ Fartlek
                             ☐ Hard

Start Energy ↑ → ↓   Recovery Energy ↑ → ↓

Duration _____   You No-Showed ☐
                             (Oops, Reset   Tomorrow)

NOTES:

SAT. /   CURRENT STREAK ___

You Showed Up/Rest Day ☐   **INTENSITY**
When? _____   ☐ Easy
Where? _____   ☐ Moderate/Zone2
Activity _____   ☐ Fartlek
                             ☐ Hard

Start Energy ↑ → ↓   Recovery Energy ↑ → ↓

Duration _____   You No-Showed ☐
                             (Oops, Reset   Tomorrow)

NOTES:

SUN. / CURRENT STREAK ___

You Showed Up/Rest Day ☐
When? _____
Where? _____
Activity _____

INTENSITY
☐ Easy
☐ Moderate/Zone2
☐ Fartlek
☐ Hard

Start Energy ↑ → ↓

Duration _____

Recovery Energy ↑ → ↓

You No-Showed ☐
(Oops, Reset Tomorrow)

NOTES:

WEEKLY SUMMARY

CURRENT STREAK ___
RECORD STREAK ___

Total Days You Showed Up/Rest Days _____
Total Days You No-Showed _____
Total Exercise Time _____
Weekly Step Avg. _____

NOTES:

WEEK 3.

MON. / CURRENT STREAK ___

You Showed Up/Rest Day ☐   **INTENSITY**
When? _____   ☐ Easy
Where? _____   ☐ Moderate/Zone2
Activity _____   ☐ Fartlek
                             ☐ Hard

Start Energy ↑ → ↓   Recovery Energy ↑ → ↓

Duration _____   You No-Showed ☐
                             (Oops, Reset   Tomorrow)

NOTES:

TUE. / CURRENT STREAK ___

You Showed Up/Rest Day ☐   **INTENSITY**
When? _____   ☐ Easy
Where? _____   ☐ Moderate/Zone2
Activity _____   ☐ Fartlek
                             ☐ Hard

Start Energy ↑ → ↓   Recovery Energy ↑ → ↓

Duration _____   You No-Showed ☐
                             (Oops, Reset   Tomorrow)

NOTES:

WED. / CURRENT STREAK ___

You Showed Up/Rest Day ☐
When? _____
Where? _____
Activity _____

INTENSITY
☐ Easy
☐ Moderate/Zone2
☐ Fartlek
☐ Hard

Start Energy ↑ → ↓

Duration _____

Recovery Energy ↑ → ↓

You No-Showed ☐
(Oops, Reset Tomorrow)

NOTES:

THU. / CURRENT STREAK ___

You Showed Up/Rest Day ☐
When? _____
Where? _____
Activity _____

INTENSITY
☐ Easy
☐ Moderate/Zone2
☐ Fartlek
☐ Hard

Start Energy ↑ → ↓

Duration _____

Recovery Energy ↑ → ↓

You No-Showed ☐
(Oops, Reset Tomorrow)

NOTES:

FRI. / CURRENT STREAK ___

You Showed Up/Rest Day ☐   **INTENSITY**
When? _____   ☐ Easy
Where? _____   ☐ Moderate/Zone2
Activity _____   ☐ Fartlek
                                    ☐ Hard

Start Energy ↑ → ↓   Recovery Energy ↑ → ↓

Duration _____   You No-Showed ☐
                                    (Oops, Reset   Tomorrow)

NOTES:

SAT. / CURRENT STREAK ___

You Showed Up/Rest Day ☐   **INTENSITY**
When? _____   ☐ Easy
Where? _____   ☐ Moderate/Zone2
Activity _____   ☐ Fartlek
                                    ☐ Hard

Start Energy ↑ → ↓   Recovery Energy ↑ → ↓

Duration _____   You No-Showed ☐
                                    (Oops, Reset   Tomorrow)

NOTES:

SUN. / CURRENT STREAK ___

You Showed Up/Rest Day ☐   **INTENSITY**

When? _____   ☐ Easy

Where? _____   ☐ Moderate/Zone2

Activity _____   ☐ Fartlek

                                     ☐ Hard

Start Energy ↑ → ↓   Recovery Energy ↑ → ↓

Duration _____   You No-Showed ☐
                                       (Oops, Reset Tomorrow)

NOTES:

WEEKLY SUMMARY

CURRENT STREAK ___

RECORD STREAK ___

Total Days You Showed Up/Rest Days _____

Total Days You No-Showed _____

Total Exercise Time _____

Weekly Step Avg. _____

NOTES:

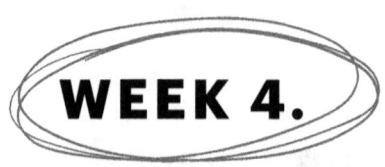

WEEK 4.

MON. / CURRENT STREAK ___

You Showed Up/Rest Day ☐
When? _____
Where? _____
Activity _____

INTENSITY
☐ Easy
☐ Moderate/Zone2
☐ Fartlek
☐ Hard

Start Energy ↑ → ↓   Recovery Energy ↑ → ↓

Duration _____
You No-Showed ☐
(Oops, Reset   Tomorrow)

NOTES:

TUE. / CURRENT STREAK ___

You Showed Up/Rest Day ☐
When? _____
Where? _____
Activity _____

INTENSITY
☐ Easy
☐ Moderate/Zone2
☐ Fartlek
☐ Hard

Start Energy ↑ → ↓   Recovery Energy ↑ → ↓

Duration _____
You No-Showed ☐
(Oops, Reset   Tomorrow)

NOTES:

WED. / CURRENT STREAK ___

You Showed Up/Rest Day ☐
When? _____
Where? _____
Activity _____

INTENSITY
☐ Easy
☐ Moderate/Zone2
☐ Fartlek
☐ Hard

Start Energy ↑ → ↓

Recovery Energy ↑ → ↓

Duration _____

You No-Showed ☐
(Oops, Reset   Tomorrow)

NOTES:

THU. / CURRENT STREAK ___

You Showed Up/Rest Day ☐
When? _____
Where? _____
Activity _____

INTENSITY
☐ Easy
☐ Moderate/Zone2
☐ Fartlek
☐ Hard

Start Energy ↑ → ↓

Recovery Energy ↑ → ↓

Duration _____

You No-Showed ☐
(Oops, Reset   Tomorrow)

NOTES:

FRI. /   CURRENT STREAK ___

You Showed Up/Rest Day ☐   **INTENSITY**
When? _____   ☐ Easy
Where? _____   ☐ Moderate/Zone2
Activity _____   ☐ Fartlek
                                  ☐ Hard

Start Energy ↑ → ↓   Recovery Energy ↑ → ↓

Duration _____   You No-Showed ☐
                                (Oops, Reset   Tomorrow)

NOTES:

SAT. /   CURRENT STREAK ___

You Showed Up/Rest Day ☐   **INTENSITY**
When? _____   ☐ Easy
Where? _____   ☐ Moderate/Zone2
Activity _____   ☐ Fartlek
                                  ☐ Hard

Start Energy ↑ → ↓   Recovery Energy ↑ → ↓

Duration _____   You No-Showed ☐
                                (Oops, Reset   Tomorrow)

NOTES:

SUN. / CURRENT STREAK ___

You Showed Up/Rest Day ☐
When? _____
Where? _____
Activity _____

INTENSITY
☐ Easy
☐ Moderate/Zone2
☐ Fartlek
☐ Hard

Start Energy ↑ → ↓

Duration _____

Recovery Energy ↑ → ↓

You No-Showed ☐
(Oops, Reset Tomorrow)

NOTES:

WEEKLY SUMMARY

CURRENT STREAK ___
RECORD STREAK ___

Total Days You Showed Up/Rest Days _____
Total Days You No-Showed _____
Total Exercise Time _____
Weekly Step Avg. _____

NOTES:

MONTHLY SUMMARY

CURRENT STREAK _____

RECORD STREAK _____

Total Days You Showed Up/Rest Days _____

Total Days You No-Showed _____

Almost Consistent Win Rate % _____
(e.g. 2 No-Shows in 30 Day Month=28. Then 28÷30=93%)

Monthly Step Avg. _____

NOTES:

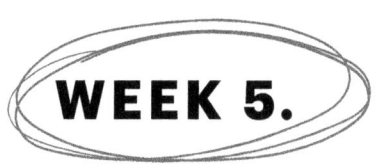

WEEK 5.

MON. / CURRENT STREAK ___

You Showed Up/Rest Day ☐
When? _____
Where? _____
Activity _____

INTENSITY
☐ Easy
☐ Moderate/Zone2
☐ Fartlek
☐ Hard

Start Energy ↑ → ↓   Recovery Energy ↑ → ↓

Duration _____   You No-Showed ☐
(Oops, Reset Tomorrow)

NOTES:

TUE. / CURRENT STREAK ___

You Showed Up/Rest Day ☐
When? _____
Where? _____
Activity _____

INTENSITY
☐ Easy
☐ Moderate/Zone2
☐ Fartlek
☐ Hard

Start Energy ↑ → ↓   Recovery Energy ↑ → ↓

Duration _____   You No-Showed ☐
(Oops, Reset Tomorrow)

NOTES:

WED. / CURRENT STREAK ___

You Showed Up/Rest Day ☐   **INTENSITY**
When? _____   ☐ Easy
Where? _____   ☐ Moderate/Zone2
Activity _____   ☐ Fartlek
                                  ☐ Hard

Start Energy ↑ → ↓   Recovery Energy ↑ → ↓

Duration _____   You No-Showed ☐
                                  (Oops, Reset   Tomorrow)

NOTES:

THU. / CURRENT STREAK ___

You Showed Up/Rest Day ☐   **INTENSITY**
When? _____   ☐ Easy
Where? _____   ☐ Moderate/Zone2
Activity _____   ☐ Fartlek
                                  ☐ Hard

Start Energy ↑ → ↓   Recovery Energy ↑ → ↓

Duration _____   You No-Showed ☐
                                  (Oops, Reset   Tomorrow)

NOTES:

FRI. /   CURRENT STREAK ___

You Showed Up/Rest Day ☐   **INTENSITY**
When? _____   ☐ Easy
Where? _____   ☐ Moderate/Zone2
Activity _____   ☐ Fartlek
                                              ☐ Hard

Start Energy ↑ → ↓   Recovery Energy ↑ → ↓

Duration _____   You No-Showed ☐
                                              (Oops, Reset   Tomorrow)

NOTES:

SAT. /   CURRENT STREAK ___

You Showed Up/Rest Day ☐   **INTENSITY**
When? _____   ☐ Easy
Where? _____   ☐ Moderate/Zone2
Activity _____   ☐ Fartlek
                                              ☐ Hard

Start Energy ↑ → ↓   Recovery Energy ↑ → ↓

Duration _____   You No-Showed ☐
                                              (Oops, Reset   Tomorrow)

NOTES:

SUN. / CURRENT STREAK ___

You Showed Up/Rest Day ☐   **INTENSITY**
When? _____   ☐ Easy
Where? _____   ☐ Moderate/Zone2
Activity _____   ☐ Fartlek
                              ☐ Hard

Start Energy ↑ → ↓   Recovery Energy ↑ → ↓
Duration _____   You No-Showed ☐
                              (Oops, Reset Tomorrow)

NOTES:

WEEKLY SUMMARY

CURRENT STREAK ___
RECORD STREAK ___

Total Days You Showed Up/Rest Days _____
Total Days You No-Showed _____
Total Exercise Time _____
Weekly Step Avg. _____

NOTES:

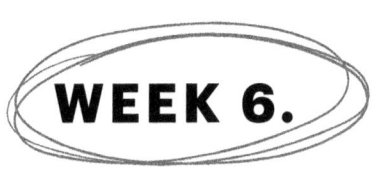

WEEK 6.

MON. / CURRENT STREAK ___

You Showed Up/Rest Day ☐ **INTENSITY**
When? _____ ☐ Easy
Where? _____ ☐ Moderate/Zone2
Activity _____ ☐ Fartlek
☐ Hard

Start Energy ↑ → ↓   Recovery Energy ↑ → ↓

Duration _____ You No-Showed ☐
(Oops, Reset Tomorrow)

NOTES:

TUE. / CURRENT STREAK ___

You Showed Up/Rest Day ☐ **INTENSITY**
When? _____ ☐ Easy
Where? _____ ☐ Moderate/Zone2
Activity _____ ☐ Fartlek
☐ Hard

Start Energy ↑ → ↓   Recovery Energy ↑ → ↓

Duration _____ You No-Showed ☐
(Oops, Reset Tomorrow)

NOTES:

WED. / CURRENT STREAK ___

You Showed Up/Rest Day ☐   **INTENSITY**
When? _____   ☐ Easy
Where? _____   ☐ Moderate/Zone2
Activity _____   ☐ Fartlek
                              ☐ Hard

Start Energy ↑ → ↓   Recovery Energy ↑ → ↓

Duration _____   You No-Showed ☐
                              (Oops, Reset   Tomorrow)

NOTES:

THU. / CURRENT STREAK ___

You Showed Up/Rest Day ☐   **INTENSITY**
When? _____   ☐ Easy
Where? _____   ☐ Moderate/Zone2
Activity _____   ☐ Fartlek
                              ☐ Hard

Start Energy ↑ → ↓   Recovery Energy ↑ → ↓

Duration _____   You No-Showed ☐
                              (Oops, Reset   Tomorrow)

NOTES:

FRI. / CURRENT STREAK ___

You Showed Up/Rest Day ☐
When? _____
Where? _____
Activity _____

INTENSITY
☐ Easy
☐ Moderate/Zone2
☐ Fartlek
☐ Hard

Start Energy ↑ → ↓
Duration _____

Recovery Energy ↑ → ↓
You No-Showed ☐
(Oops, Reset   Tomorrow)

NOTES:

SAT. / CURRENT STREAK ___

You Showed Up/Rest Day ☐
When? _____
Where? _____
Activity _____

INTENSITY
☐ Easy
☐ Moderate/Zone2
☐ Fartlek
☐ Hard

Start Energy ↑ → ↓
Duration _____

Recovery Energy ↑ → ↓
You No-Showed ☐
(Oops, Reset   Tomorrow)

NOTES:

SUN. / CURRENT STREAK ____

You Showed Up/Rest Day ☐   **INTENSITY**
When? _____   ☐ Easy
Where? _____   ☐ Moderate/Zone2
Activity _____ ☐ Fartlek
                            ☐ Hard

Start Energy ↑ → ↓   Recovery Energy ↑ → ↓

Duration _____ You No-Showed ☐
                            (Oops, Reset   Tomorrow)

NOTES:

WEEKLY SUMMARY

CURRENT STREAK ____
RECORD STREAK ____

Total Days You Showed Up/Rest Days _____
Total Days You No-Showed _____
Total Exercise Time _____
Weekly Step Avg. _____

NOTES:

WEEK 7.

MON. / CURRENT STREAK ___

You Showed Up/Rest Day ☐   **INTENSITY**
When? _____   ☐ Easy
Where? _____ ☐ Moderate/Zone2
Activity _____ ☐ Fartlek
                             ☐ Hard

Start Energy ↑ → ↓   Recovery Energy ↑ → ↓

Duration _____ You No-Showed ☐
                            (Oops, Reset   Tomorrow)

NOTES:

TUE. / CURRENT STREAK ___

You Showed Up/Rest Day ☐   **INTENSITY**
When? _____   ☐ Easy
Where? _____ ☐ Moderate/Zone2
Activity _____ ☐ Fartlek
                             ☐ Hard

Start Energy ↑ → ↓   Recovery Energy ↑ → ↓

Duration _____ You No-Showed ☐
                            (Oops, Reset   Tomorrow)

NOTES:

WED. / CURRENT STREAK ___

You Showed Up/Rest Day ☐   **INTENSITY**
When? _____   ☐ Easy
Where? _____   ☐ Moderate/Zone2
Activity _____   ☐ Fartlek
                                                 ☐ Hard

Start Energy ↑ → ↓   Recovery Energy ↑ → ↓

Duration _____   You No-Showed ☐
                                                 (Oops, Reset   Tomorrow)

NOTES:

THU. / CURRENT STREAK ___

You Showed Up/Rest Day ☐   **INTENSITY**
When? _____   ☐ Easy
Where? _____   ☐ Moderate/Zone2
Activity _____   ☐ Fartlek
                                                 ☐ Hard

Start Energy ↑ → ↓   Recovery Energy ↑ → ↓

Duration _____   You No-Showed ☐
                                                 (Oops, Reset   Tomorrow)

NOTES:

FRI. /   CURRENT STREAK ____

You Showed Up/Rest Day ☐
When? _____
Where? _____
Activity _____

INTENSITY
☐ Easy
☐ Moderate/Zone2
☐ Fartlek
☐ Hard

Start Energy ↑ → ↓

Duration _____

Recovery Energy ↑ → ↓

You No-Showed ☐
(Oops, Reset   Tomorrow)

NOTES:

SAT. /   CURRENT STREAK ____

You Showed Up/Rest Day ☐
When? _____
Where? _____
Activity _____

INTENSITY
☐ Easy
☐ Moderate/Zone2
☐ Fartlek
☐ Hard

Start Energy ↑ → ↓

Duration _____

Recovery Energy ↑ → ↓

You No-Showed ☐
(Oops, Reset   Tomorrow)

NOTES:

SUN. / CURRENT STREAK ____

You Showed Up/Rest Day ☐   **INTENSITY**
When? _____   ☐ Easy
Where? _____   ☐ Moderate/Zone2
Activity _____   ☐ Fartlek
    ☐ Hard

Start Energy ↑ → ↓   Recovery Energy ↑ → ↓
Duration _____   You No-Showed ☐
    (Oops, Reset   Tomorrow)

NOTES:

WEEKLY SUMMARY

CURRENT STREAK _____
RECORD STREAK _____
Total Days You Showed Up/Rest Days _____
Total Days You No-Showed _____
Total Exercise Time _____
Weekly Step Avg. _____

NOTES:

WEEK 8.

MON. / CURRENT STREAK ____

You Showed Up/Rest Day ☐ **INTENSITY**
When? _____ ☐ Easy
Where? _____ ☐ Moderate/Zone2
Activity _____ ☐ Fartlek
☐ Hard

Start Energy ↑ → ↓   Recovery Energy ↑ → ↓

Duration _____ You No-Showed ☐
(Oops, Reset   Tomorrow)

NOTES:

TUE. / CURRENT STREAK ____

You Showed Up/Rest Day ☐ **INTENSITY**
When? _____ ☐ Easy
Where? _____ ☐ Moderate/Zone2
Activity _____ ☐ Fartlek
☐ Hard

Start Energy ↑ → ↓   Recovery Energy ↑ → ↓

Duration _____ You No-Showed ☐
(Oops, Reset   Tomorrow)

NOTES:

WED. / CURRENT STREAK ___

You Showed Up/Rest Day ☐   **INTENSITY**
When? _____   ☐ Easy
Where? _____   ☐ Moderate/Zone2
Activity _____   ☐ Fartlek
☐ Hard

Start Energy ↑ → ↓   Recovery Energy ↑ → ↓

Duration _____   You No-Showed ☐
(Oops, Reset   Tomorrow)

NOTES:

THU. / CURRENT STREAK ___

You Showed Up/Rest Day ☐   **INTENSITY**
When? _____   ☐ Easy
Where? _____   ☐ Moderate/Zone2
Activity _____   ☐ Fartlek
☐ Hard

Start Energy ↑ → ↓   Recovery Energy ↑ → ↓

Duration _____   You No-Showed ☐
(Oops, Reset   Tomorrow)

NOTES:

FRI. / CURRENT STREAK ___

You Showed Up/Rest Day ☐
When? _____
Where? _____
Activity _____

INTENSITY
☐ Easy
☐ Moderate/Zone2
☐ Fartlek
☐ Hard

Start Energy ↑ → ↓

Recovery Energy ↑ → ↓

Duration _____

You No-Showed ☐
(Oops, Reset Tomorrow)

NOTES:

SAT. / CURRENT STREAK ___

You Showed Up/Rest Day ☐
When? _____
Where? _____
Activity _____

INTENSITY
☐ Easy
☐ Moderate/Zone2
☐ Fartlek
☐ Hard

Start Energy ↑ → ↓

Recovery Energy ↑ → ↓

Duration _____

You No-Showed ☐
(Oops, Reset Tomorrow)

NOTES:

SUN. / CURRENT STREAK ____

You Showed Up/Rest Day ☐   **INTENSITY**
When? _____   ☐ Easy
Where? _____   ☐ Moderate/Zone2
Activity _____   ☐ Fartlek
                            ☐ Hard

Start Energy ↑ → ↓   Recovery Energy ↑ → ↓
Duration _____   You No-Showed ☐
                           (Oops, Reset   Tomorrow)

NOTES:

WEEKLY SUMMARY

CURRENT STREAK ____
RECORD STREAK ____

Total Days You Showed Up/Rest Days _____
Total Days You No-Showed _____
Total Exercise Time _____
Weekly Step Avg. _____

NOTES:

MONTHLY SUMMARY

CURRENT STREAK ____
RECORD STREAK ____

Total Days You Showed Up/Rest Days _____

Total Days You No-Showed _____

Almost Consistent Win Rate % _____
(e.g. 2 No-Shows in 30 Day Month=28. Then 28÷30=93%)

Monthly Step Avg. _____

NOTES:

WEEK 9.

MON. / CURRENT STREAK ___

You Showed Up/Rest Day ☐   **INTENSITY**
When? _____   ☐ Easy
Where? _____   ☐ Moderate/Zone2
Activity _____   ☐ Fartlek
                               ☐ Hard

Start Energy ↑ → ↓   Recovery Energy ↑ → ↓

Duration _____   You No-Showed ☐
                             (Oops, Reset   Tomorrow)

NOTES:

TUE. / CURRENT STREAK ___

You Showed Up/Rest Day ☐   **INTENSITY**
When? _____   ☐ Easy
Where? _____   ☐ Moderate/Zone2
Activity _____   ☐ Fartlek
                               ☐ Hard

Start Energy ↑ → ↓   Recovery Energy ↑ → ↓

Duration _____   You No-Showed ☐
                             (Oops, Reset   Tomorrow)

NOTES:

WED. / CURRENT STREAK ___

You Showed Up/Rest Day ☐
When? _____
Where? _____
Activity _____

INTENSITY
☐ Easy
☐ Moderate/Zone2
☐ Fartlek
☐ Hard

Start Energy ↑ → ↓

Recovery Energy ↑ → ↓

Duration _____

You No-Showed ☐
(Oops, Reset Tomorrow)

NOTES:

THU. / CURRENT STREAK ___

You Showed Up/Rest Day ☐
When? _____
Where? _____
Activity _____

INTENSITY
☐ Easy
☐ Moderate/Zone2
☐ Fartlek
☐ Hard

Start Energy ↑ → ↓

Recovery Energy ↑ → ↓

Duration _____

You No-Showed ☐
(Oops, Reset Tomorrow)

NOTES:

FRI. /   CURRENT STREAK ___

You Showed Up/Rest Day ☐   **INTENSITY**
When? _____   ☐ Easy
Where? _____   ☐ Moderate/Zone2
Activity _____   ☐ Fartlek
                              ☐ Hard

Start Energy ↑ → ↓   Recovery Energy ↑ → ↓

Duration _____   You No-Showed ☐
                            (Oops, Reset   Tomorrow)

NOTES:

SAT. /   CURRENT STREAK ___

You Showed Up/Rest Day ☐   **INTENSITY**
When? _____   ☐ Easy
Where? _____   ☐ Moderate/Zone2
Activity _____   ☐ Fartlek
                              ☐ Hard

Start Energy ↑ → ↓   Recovery Energy ↑ → ↓

Duration _____   You No-Showed ☐
                            (Oops, Reset   Tomorrow)

NOTES:

SUN. / CURRENT STREAK ____

You Showed Up/Rest Day ☐

When? _____

Where? _____

Activity _____

INTENSITY
- ☐ Easy
- ☐ Moderate/Zone2
- ☐ Fartlek
- ☐ Hard

Start Energy ↑ → ↓

Duration _____

Recovery Energy ↑ → ↓

You No-Showed ☐
(Oops, Reset Tomorrow)

NOTES:

WEEKLY SUMMARY

CURRENT STREAK ____

RECORD STREAK ____

Total Days You Showed Up/Rest Days _____

Total Days You No-Showed _____

Total Exercise Time _____

Weekly Step Avg. _____

NOTES:

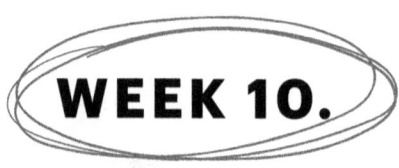
WEEK 10.

MON. / CURRENT STREAK ___

You Showed Up/Rest Day ☐   **INTENSITY**
When? _____   ☐ Easy
Where? _____   ☐ Moderate/Zone2
Activity _____   ☐ Fartlek
   ☐ Hard

Start Energy ↑ → ↓   Recovery Energy ↑ → ↓

Duration _____   You No-Showed ☐
   (Oops, Reset Tomorrow)

NOTES:

TUE. / CURRENT STREAK ___

You Showed Up/Rest Day ☐   **INTENSITY**
When? _____   ☐ Easy
Where? _____   ☐ Moderate/Zone2
Activity _____   ☐ Fartlek
   ☐ Hard

Start Energy ↑ → ↓   Recovery Energy ↑ → ↓

Duration _____   You No-Showed ☐
   (Oops, Reset Tomorrow)

NOTES:

WED. / CURRENT STREAK ___

You Showed Up/Rest Day ☐
When? _____
Where? _____
Activity _____

INTENSITY
☐ Easy
☐ Moderate/Zone2
☐ Fartlek
☐ Hard

Start Energy ↑ → ↓

Recovery Energy ↑ → ↓

Duration _____

You No-Showed ☐
(Oops, Reset   Tomorrow)

NOTES:

THU. / CURRENT STREAK ___

You Showed Up/Rest Day ☐
When? _____
Where? _____
Activity _____

INTENSITY
☐ Easy
☐ Moderate/Zone2
☐ Fartlek
☐ Hard

Start Energy ↑ → ↓

Recovery Energy ↑ → ↓

Duration _____

You No-Showed ☐
(Oops, Reset   Tomorrow)

NOTES:

FRI. / CURRENT STREAK ____

You Showed Up/Rest Day ☐   **INTENSITY**
When? _____   ☐ Easy
Where? _____   ☐ Moderate/Zone2
Activity _____   ☐ Fartlek
                                 ☐ Hard

Start Energy ↑ → ↓   Recovery Energy ↑ → ↓

Duration _____   You No-Showed ☐
                                 (Oops, Reset   Tomorrow)

NOTES:

SAT. / CURRENT STREAK ____

You Showed Up/Rest Day ☐   **INTENSITY**
When? _____   ☐ Easy
Where? _____   ☐ Moderate/Zone2
Activity _____   ☐ Fartlek
                                 ☐ Hard

Start Energy ↑ → ↓   Recovery Energy ↑ → ↓

Duration _____   You No-Showed ☐
                                 (Oops, Reset   Tomorrow)

NOTES:

SUN. / CURRENT STREAK ___

You Showed Up/Rest Day ☐
When? _____
Where? _____
Activity _____

INTENSITY
☐ Easy
☐ Moderate/Zone2
☐ Fartlek
☐ Hard

Start Energy ↑ → ↓

Duration _____

Recovery Energy ↑ → ↓

You No-Showed ☐
(Oops, Reset Tomorrow)

NOTES:

WEEKLY SUMMARY

CURRENT STREAK ___

RECORD STREAK ___

Total Days You Showed Up/Rest Days _____
Total Days You No-Showed _____
Total Exercise Time _____
Weekly Step Avg. _____

NOTES:

WEEK 11.

MON. / CURRENT STREAK ___

You Showed Up/Rest Day ☐   **INTENSITY**
When? _____   ☐ Easy
Where? _____   ☐ Moderate/Zone2
Activity _____   ☐ Fartlek
   ☐ Hard

Start Energy ↑ → ↓   Recovery Energy ↑ → ↓

Duration _____   You No-Showed ☐
(Oops, Reset Tomorrow)

NOTES:

TUE. / CURRENT STREAK ___

You Showed Up/Rest Day ☐   **INTENSITY**
When? _____   ☐ Easy
Where? _____   ☐ Moderate/Zone2
Activity _____   ☐ Fartlek
   ☐ Hard

Start Energy ↑ → ↓   Recovery Energy ↑ → ↓

Duration _____   You No-Showed ☐
(Oops, Reset Tomorrow)

NOTES:

WED. / CURRENT STREAK ___

You Showed Up/Rest Day ☐   **INTENSITY**
When? _____   ☐ Easy
Where? _____   ☐ Moderate/Zone2
Activity _____   ☐ Fartlek
                                  ☐ Hard

Start Energy ↑ → ↓   Recovery Energy ↑ → ↓

Duration _____   You No-Showed ☐
                                  (Oops, Reset Tomorrow)

NOTES:

THU. / CURRENT STREAK ___

You Showed Up/Rest Day ☐   **INTENSITY**
When? _____   ☐ Easy
Where? _____   ☐ Moderate/Zone2
Activity _____   ☐ Fartlek
                                  ☐ Hard

Start Energy ↑ → ↓   Recovery Energy ↑ → ↓

Duration _____   You No-Showed ☐
                                  (Oops, Reset Tomorrow)

NOTES:

FRI. / CURRENT STREAK ___

You Showed Up/Rest Day ☐   **INTENSITY**
When? _____   ☐ Easy
Where? _____   ☐ Moderate/Zone2
Activity _____ ☐ Fartlek
                             ☐ Hard

Start Energy ↑ → ↓   Recovery Energy ↑ → ↓

Duration _____ You No-Showed ☐
                             (Oops, Reset   Tomorrow)

NOTES:

SAT. / CURRENT STREAK ___

You Showed Up/Rest Day ☐   **INTENSITY**
When? _____   ☐ Easy
Where? _____   ☐ Moderate/Zone2
Activity _____ ☐ Fartlek
                             ☐ Hard

Start Energy ↑ → ↓   Recovery Energy ↑ → ↓

Duration _____ You No-Showed ☐
                             (Oops, Reset   Tomorrow)

NOTES:

SUN. / CURRENT STREAK ___

You Showed Up/Rest Day ☐
When? _____
Where? _____
Activity _____

INTENSITY
☐ Easy
☐ Moderate/Zone2
☐ Fartlek
☐ Hard

Start Energy ↑ → ↓

Duration _____

Recovery Energy ↑ → ↓

You No-Showed ☐
(Oops, Reset Tomorrow)

NOTES:

WEEKLY SUMMARY

CURRENT STREAK ___
RECORD STREAK ___

Total Days You Showed Up/Rest Days _____
Total Days You No-Showed _____
Total Exercise Time _____
Weekly Step Avg. _____

NOTES:

WEEK 12.

MON. / CURRENT STREAK ___

You Showed Up/Rest Day ☐

When? _____

Where? _____

Activity _____

INTENSITY
☐ Easy
☐ Moderate/Zone2
☐ Fartlek
☐ Hard

Start Energy ↑ → ↓   Recovery Energy ↑ → ↓

Duration _____

You No-Showed ☐
(Oops, Reset Tomorrow)

NOTES:

TUE. / CURRENT STREAK ___

You Showed Up/Rest Day ☐

When? _____

Where? _____

Activity _____

INTENSITY
☐ Easy
☐ Moderate/Zone2
☐ Fartlek
☐ Hard

Start Energy ↑ → ↓   Recovery Energy ↑ → ↓

Duration _____

You No-Showed ☐
(Oops, Reset Tomorrow)

NOTES:

WED. / CURRENT STREAK ___

You Showed Up/Rest Day ☐
When? _____
Where? _____
Activity _____

INTENSITY
☐ Easy
☐ Moderate/Zone2
☐ Fartlek
☐ Hard

Start Energy ↑ → ↓

Duration _____

Recovery Energy ↑ → ↓

You No-Showed ☐
(Oops, Reset Tomorrow)

NOTES:

THU. / CURRENT STREAK ___

You Showed Up/Rest Day ☐
When? _____
Where? _____
Activity _____

INTENSITY
☐ Easy
☐ Moderate/Zone2
☐ Fartlek
☐ Hard

Start Energy ↑ → ↓

Duration _____

Recovery Energy ↑ → ↓

You No-Showed ☐
(Oops, Reset Tomorrow)

NOTES:

FRI. / CURRENT STREAK ___

You Showed Up/Rest Day ☐   **INTENSITY**
When? _____   ☐ Easy
Where? _____   ☐ Moderate/Zone2
Activity _____   ☐ Fartlek
　　　　　　　　　　　　　☐ Hard

Start Energy ↑ → ↓　　Recovery Energy ↑ → ↓

Duration _____   You No-Showed ☐
　　　　　　　　　　　　　(Oops, Reset Tomorrow)

NOTES:

SAT. / CURRENT STREAK ___

You Showed Up/Rest Day ☐   **INTENSITY**
When? _____   ☐ Easy
Where? _____   ☐ Moderate/Zone2
Activity _____   ☐ Fartlek
　　　　　　　　　　　　　☐ Hard

Start Energy ↑ → ↓　　Recovery Energy ↑ → ↓

Duration _____   You No-Showed ☐
　　　　　　　　　　　　　(Oops, Reset Tomorrow)

NOTES:

SUN. / CURRENT STREAK ___

You Showed Up/Rest Day ☐   **INTENSITY**
When? _____ ☐ Easy
Where? _____ ☐ Moderate/Zone2
Activity _____ ☐ Fartlek
                              ☐ Hard

Start Energy ↑ → ↓   Recovery Energy ↑ → ↓
Duration _____   You No-Showed ☐
                             (Oops, Reset Tomorrow)

NOTES:

WEEKLY SUMMARY

CURRENT STREAK ___
RECORD STREAK ___

Total Days You Showed Up/Rest Days _____
Total Days You No-Showed _____
Total Exercise Time _____
Weekly Step Avg. _____

NOTES:

MONTHLY SUMMARY

CURRENT STREAK _____
RECORD STREAK _____

Total Days You Showed Up/Rest Days _____

Total Days You No-Showed _____

Almost Consistent Win Rate % _____
(e.g. 2 No-Shows in 30 Day Month=28. Then 28÷30=93%)

Monthly Step Avg. _____

NOTES:

ACKNOWLEDGMENTS

Fin, Mac, Lula Mulligan, and Bubba and Poncho, two lovable ranch dogs, would stop by for a regular visit. They would look at the maze of 5x8 cards I had scattered on my desk and ask, "When's the book going to be finished?"

The pleasant nudging from my grandkids and regular conversations with my son Jeff was vital as we discussed the mental side of sports from his perspective as a racquet sports teaching professional. My interest in helping people develop positive exercise habits and his teaching approach had one thing in common: We both focused on "Process," not outcome.

I would also like to thank my daughter-in-law, Ashley Dahl, M.D., for her love, support, and review of portions of the book. Ashley proves daily that even the busiest among us can find time and prioritize Fitness.

Love and thanks to my son Sean Gale, gym owner and personal trainer, for our regular sports conversations and his thoughtful review. We have a shared passion and respect for people who keep a positive attitude and stay on course, even when things aren't perfect. No whining; just show up and do something.

I would like to thank my friends at Mayfly Design and Publishing Services for their much-needed expertise and support throughout the process. Julie and Ryan Scheife and graphic designer Molly Mortimer smoothed out all the bumps in the road.

Suzanne Coner's edit support was more than I could have hoped for. Suzanne's love of running and football and her scholarly language skills made her the perfect fit. Thank you, Suzanne.

I'm grateful and would like to acknowledge the large cast of friends, family, and coaches who've positively impacted me over the years:

My brother John and my son Jerry who have made walking a part of their lives.

Coaches Jerry Bell, Upland High School, and John Scolinos, Pepperdine University, were the finest role models a young guy could have.

Don Manoukian, Stanford University, and the Oakland Raiders. My business partner and the big brother I never had.

I've walked hundreds of miles of golf courses with my business partner and friend, Dan Stuart.

Business partners and friends, Gregg Spieker and Lee Spieker. Both have been leaders in the successful promotion of fitness for many years

John Todor, PhD, for his academic guidance and friendship.

Mike Hanamura, for his efforts as the high school student body president who never quit. He continues to keep in touch, encouraging and supporting. Mike, you are the definition of leadership.

Wendy, I carry on. Your guidance through this writing process has been palpable. I love you.

www.ingramcontent.com/pod-product-compliance
Lightning Source LLC
Chambersburg PA
CBHW070624030426
42337CB00020B/3911